THE

2003

BODY ALMANAC

Your Personal Guide to Bone and Joint Health At Any Age

AMERICAN ACADEMY OF
ORTHOPAEDIC SURGEONS

THE
2003
BODY
ALMANAC

Edited by
Glenn B. Pfeffer, MD
Ramon L. Jimenez, MD
John F. Sarwark, MD
Letha Yurko-Griffin, MD, PhD

Written by
Susan Crites Price

Published by the
American Academy of Orthopaedic Surgeons
6300 North River Road
Rosemont, IL 60018

American Academy of Orthopaedic Surgeons

Staff

Mark Wieting, *Vice President,*
Educational Programs
Marilyn L. Fox, PhD, *Director,*
Department of Publications
Lynne Roby Shindoll, *Managing Editor*
Gayle Ekblad, *Associate Senior Editor*
Mary Steermann, *Manager,*
Production and Archives
David Stanley, *Assistant Production*
Manager
Sophie Tosta, *Assistant Production*
Manager
Courtney Astle, *Production Assistant*
Karen Danca, *Production Assistant*
Laura Andujar, *Publications Assistant*

The figures on pages 17, 18, and 19 are
courtesy of Greater Milwaukee Computer
Imaging, Milwaukee, WI.

Cover Design by Tom Kepler
Book Design by David Stanley
Illustrations by Christine Young, Stacy
Lund-Levy, and Brian Stafford.

The 2003 Body Almanac
American Academy of Orthopaedic
Surgeons

First Edition
Copyright © 2003 by the
American Academy of Orthopaedic
Surgeons

ISBN 0-89203-281-2

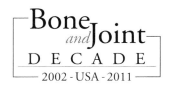

Dear Reader,

We have published the *The 2003 Body Almanac* to help you take care of yourself or someone you love. The American Academy of Orthopaedic Surgeons and its members have been devoted to the care of the musculoskeletal system for 70 years, and we know that minor aches and pains have a variety of causes; some need immediate attention while others can be treated at home. This text, developed by four orthopaedic surgeon editors, is our "top 100" list of common problems and questions you have about your musculoskeletal system and the problems you may experience.

The *Almanac* is formatted and designed for easy reference. You'll find a general topics section, plus eight sections covering specific areas of the body. Only one problem or issue is addressed per chapter and each is structured in the following way:

- A definition of the problem or condition
- The classic signs and symptoms
- How it is treated
- When to call your doctor

For most conditions, you can first try home treatment, often with simple approaches such as heat, ice, rest, simple exercises, or over-the-counter remedies. With this book we hope to take the mystery out of some of these problems and help you better understand your condition and, whenever possible, to treat it simply or to prevent it from recurring. Interesting facts concerning risk factors, history, and causes for these conditions appear throughout the book as well.

You can learn how to prepare for a doctor visit, take care of a cast, select a backpack for your children, or even choose a walker for an elderly parent. Medical terms, procedures, certain operations and medical tests, and the parts of the musculoskeletal system are defined throughout the book and in a glossary. We also invite you to visit our website (www.aaos.org/almanac) if you want even more information about some of these conditions.

The 2003 Body Almanac also includes a chapter devoted to the powers of exercise. In this chapter, we emphasize the importance of physical activity for overall health, correct techniques for keeping fit, and various types of exercise programs. More than 50 simple exercises are shown, including sports warm-up/stretching, range of motion, and strengthening programs for various parts of the body.

Whether you are a soccer mom, weekend athlete, active senior, or someone in between, *The 2003 Body Almanac* is a valuable resource. We hope that with this book, you will truly have "a leg up" next time you feel a twinge in the foot or a kink in the neck.

William Tipton, MD
Executive Vice President
American Academy of Orthopaedic Surgeons

TABLE OF CONTENTS

KEEPING YOUR BODY TUNED UP

SHOULDER

ELBOW AND FOREARM

HAND AND WRIST

HIP AND THIGH

KNEE AND LOWER LEG

NECK AND SPINE

,

KEEPING YOUR BODY TUNED UP

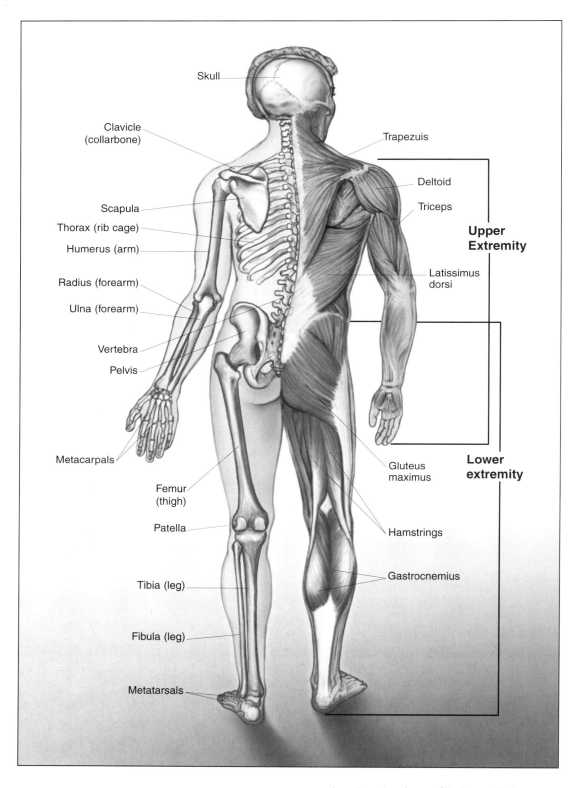

Skull

Clavicle
(collarbone)

Scapula

Thorax (rib cage)

Humerus (arm)

Radius (forearm)

Ulna (forearm)

Vertebra

Pelvis

Metacarpals

Femur
(thigh)

Patella

Tibia (leg)

Fibula (leg)

Metatarsals

Trapezuis

Deltoid

Triceps

**Upper
Extremity**

Latissimus
dorsi

**Lower
extremity**

Gluteus
maximus

Hamstrings

Gastrocnemius

KEEPING YOUR BODY TUNED UP

DID YOU EVER WISH YOUR body came with an owner's manual? It would really be handy when something goes wrong, and you are trying to decide whether you can fix it yourself or need to see a professional. If you try the do-it-yourself approach first, it would be great to have step-by-step directions. Most important, a manual could tell you how to perform preventive maintenance to avoid breakdowns in the first place. This is that book—a body almanac for your musculoskeletal system.

Whether you are an athlete or a couch potato, a toddler, an adolescent or senior citizen, you inevitably have an occasional musculoskeletal problem even if it's just a minor ache after vigorous activity or a sprain from tripping on the sidewalk. Only the rare person has never had a broken bone.

The musculoskeletal system is a wondrous thing. It's what makes humans able to walk upright, sit, stand, jump, climb, throw, and dance. Just consider one body part—the hands—and their enormous range of movement that allows humans to do everything from play the piano to perform brain surgery.

YOUR MUSCULOSKELETAL SYSTEM

The musculoskeletal system includes the body's bones, joints, ligaments, tendons, muscles, and nerves.

The bones are the body's framework. But they can't move themselves; that is the work of the muscles. These two systems working together make movement possible. An injury to either a muscle or a bone can stop movement. Fortunately, both systems are living tissues that can repair and regenerate themselves. Bones grow new bone tissue to repair a crack. Muscles can become stronger and more flexible with proper exercise.

There are 206 bones in the human body. Since bones are hard and don't bend, a series of joints where bones meet allow body parts to bend. There are several types of joints. Two of the most important for movement and which are more prone to injury are the ball-and-socket joint and the hinge joint. The ball-and-socket joint permits the widest range of motion. Examples of these are the shoulder and the hip. Hinge joints are found in the knee, ankle, fingers, and toes.

Bones don't move by themselves. That's the work of more than 650 skeletal muscles, which receive signals from the brain through nerves and respond by lengthening or shortening (flexing or stretching) to move a particular body part in the direction you want it to go.

Muscles are attached to the bones by tendons, tough bands of tissue. Ligaments are made of similarly tough tissue, and their job is to hold bones together. If you've heard it said that someone is double jointed because they can move in ways most people can't,

Know Your Parts!

- **Bones** (206 total)—give us form, upright posture, and protect our organs

- **Muscles** (650+)—help us move, breathe, and pump blood to our body

- **Joints** (ball and socket, hinge)—allow movement when two bones meet

- **Ligaments**—hold bones together

- **Tendons**—attach muscles to bones

- **Cartilage**—cushioning material attached to ends of bones

- **Bursae**—fluid-filled sacs between tendons and bones

they don't really have extra joints. They just have very flexible ligaments!

Two other structures that sometimes cause us problems are cartilage and bursae. Cartilage is the cushioning material attached to the ends of bones that reduces friction. It can wear away with age or overuse, causing pain and inflammation. Bursae are small, fluid-filled sacs that reduce friction between a tendon and a bone. A bursa can become sore with overuse, too.

Common Injuries

Much of what you'll find in *The 2003 Body Almanac* is descriptions of common injuries, what to do about them, and how to prevent them. The following list describes some common terms you will find. In addition, there is a glossary of common musculoskeletal terms in the back of the book.

1. **Sprain**—stretching or tearing a ligament
2. **Strain**—stretching or tearing a muscle or tendon
3. **Dislocation**—when the joint moves out of its proper place
4. **Simple fracture**—when the bone cracks but stays aligned
5. **Compound fracture**—when the bone cracks and the parts move apart, typically breaking the skin
6. **Stress fracture**—a common overuse injury characterized by a microscopic crack in the bone that will heal if the body part is allowed to rest while new bone growth forms
7. **Occult fracture**—a small break in the bone that may not show up on X-rays (the word occult means hidden) but may be detectable on a bone scan

Keeping Moving!

The great thing about bones and muscles is that the more you use them, the better they work. . .as long as you don't overdo it.

Muscles waste away (atrophy) when they aren't used. That's why even when you sustain an injury such as a broken bone, doctors recommend gentle exercises to keep the muscles from weakening while the bone heals. Weight-bearing exercises such as walking helps keep bones strong. Sit around too much and the bones can become brittle.

The right kinds of exercise can keep your musculoskeletal system working well, even into old age. Health-conscious baby boomers will be the models for how we don't have to become frail and stooped in later years, unlike the elderly of previous generations.

Good muscle tone is a key to preventing injury. If the muscles around the knee joint are properly conditioned, for example, you're much less likely to suffer a dislocation or ligament tear. Muscles need both stretching exercises to keep them flexible and conditioning exercises to keep them strong. (See p 22 for details on exercising for bone and muscle fitness.)

Forget "No Pain, No Gain"

A major cause of injury is jumping into a vigorous training program or a new sport without preparation. If you want to increase the level of your workout or undertake one for the first time, start at beginning levels and increase your intensity gradually.

At the beginning of every exercise session, do your muscles a favor: warm them up just like you would a car engine. A few minutes of stretching increases blood flow and helps prevent injuries from sudden demands on the muscles. A few minutes of cooldown exercises at the end of a workout helps prevent stiffness and soreness.

Listen to your body. If anything starts to hurt, stop the activity because this is a sign of injury. After the pain goes away, resume your routine gradually. The worst thing you can do is play through pain because what started out as a minor injury can become a lot worse.

Remember that you can overdo other activities as well. A day spent weeding the garden or painting the bedroom when you haven't used those muscles in a long time will almost inevitably cause aches and pains. Break the job into smaller tasks and do them over time if you aren't in good shape.

Learn Proper Technique

There are right ways and wrong ways to exercise or play a sport. Learning the proper way to pivot or land a jump, for example, goes a long way toward preventing sports injuries.

There's a proper technique for lifting a heavy load, too. If you power the lift through your legs rather than put all the strain on your back, you can avoid a backache or worse.

Remember RICE

One of the most common treatments for the conditions described in *The 2003 Body Almanac* is called RICE. This stands for Rest, Ice, Compression, and Elevation. Here's how it works:

1. **Rest.** Stop the activity that is aggravating the body part.
2. **Ice.** Apply an ice pack to reduce swelling and inflam-

mation. You can use a commercially available product, a bag of frozen vegetables, or wrap ice cubes in a towel, but don't put ice directly on your skin because that can cause frostbite.

3. **Compression.** Wrap the injured area in an elastic bandage to reduce swelling. Just don't wrap so tightly that you inhibit circulation.

4. **Elevate.** Keep the body part elevated, above the heart if possible. If the injury is to your knee, for example, lie down with your knee propped up on pillows.

Shoes and Other Equipment

A major cause of foot, ankle, and knee injuries is working out in athletic shoes that don't provide proper support. And even if the shoes worked fine when you bought them, they won't prevent injury once they are worn out. If you walk or run regularly, buy a new pair at least every year, and more often if you run more than 10 miles a week. Dress shoes can also cause problems if you wear high heels for long periods or shoes that are too tight for the shape of your feet. (See p 234 for advice on buying all types of shoes.)

If you play a sport that calls for protective equipment, always wear it in both practices and games. Anything that takes the

Exercise Essentials

1. *Warm up*
2. *Use proper technique*
3. *Start slow and increase your workout gradually*
4. *Don't ignore pain*
5. *Wear the right shoes*
6. *Drink water to stay hydrated*

stress off your bones and muscles—knee pads for gardeners, wrist pads for computer users—can help prevent problems.

Lifestyle Issues

Other factors besides exercise affect the strength of your bones and muscles. Diet is a big part of that, especially consuming adequate levels of calcium, which are critical for bone growth. The "Healthy Bones Diet" is presented on p 19.

Focusing on exercise and diet to stave off obesity can help prevent problems with knees, legs, feet, and hips that bear the brunt of the body's weight.

You may be surprised to learn that smoking is bad for bones. Along with the many other medical problems smoking causes, it's been shown to decrease bone mineral, resulting in bones that are fragile and more susceptible to fracture. Smoking also decreases blood flow to the extremities, which makes the tissues less healthy. Smokers who need surgery to correct bone or muscle problems don't recover as easily as nonsmokers.

YOUR MUSCULOSKELETAL TEAM

Orthopaedic Surgeons

Orthopaedists, also known as orthopaedic surgeons, are medical doctors (MDs) who specialize in the diagnosis, treatment (both nonsurgical and surgical), rehabilitation, and prevention of injuries and diseases of the musculoskeletal system—the bones, joints, ligaments, tendons, muscles, and nerves.

Some orthopaedists have a general practice while others specialize in treating the foot, hand, shoulder, spine, hip, knee, or more than one of these. Pediatric orthopaedists treat children, and some orthopaedists specialize in sports medicine.

Orthopaedists typically complete 14 years of formal education, including 4 years at a college or university, 4 years in medical school, 5 in an orthopaedic residency at a major medical center, and 1 optional year of specialized education. Continuing education courses keep them up to date on the many technological and treatment advances in the field.

Physical Therapists (PTs) and PT Assistants

As part of your treatment, your orthopaedic surgeon may refer you to a physical therapist. A PT helps patients relieve pain and regain function through therapeutic exercise and other techniques. (For a discussion of physical therapy methods, see p 61.) All are college graduates, most of whom earn master's degrees, and some have advanced certification in a clinical specialty.

PT assistants are skilled health care providers who work under the supervision of a PT. An assistant must complete a 2-year associate degree and is required by more than half the states to be licensed.

Occupational Therapists (OTs) and OT Assistants (OTA)

Occupational therapists assist people who, because of injury or illness, are unable to perform the tasks of daily life such as eating and bathing. They help people regain the skills needed for independent functioning, and when those skills can't be improved, they train patients in the use of adaptive equipment. They also evaluate patients' homes and office environments and recommend adaptations. They often work in tandem with PTs.

OTs complete either a bachelor's or a master's degree and must pass a national certification exam. They are regulated in all 50 states. An OTA has a 2-year degree and works under the supervision of an OT.

Athletic Trainers

Athletic trainers help athletes prevent injuries or recover from them. Some of their duties include ensuring that proper safety equipment is used, administering first aid, wrapping or bracing injured body parts, and teaching strength and flexibility exercises. A certified athletic trainer has, at minimum, earned a bachelor's degree with classroom training in sports medicine as well as clinical experience and has passed a national certification exam developed by the National Athletic Trainers' Association.

COMPLEMENTARY AND ALTERNATIVE MEDICINE PROVIDERS

Massage Therapists

Some patients turn to therapeutic massage for painful conditions. At least 30 states require massage therapists to be licensed. The National Certification Board for Therapeutic Massage and Bodywork administers a certification program. The American Massage Therapy Association requires members to complete at least 500 hours of course work at a school approved by the Commission on Massage Therapy Accreditation. Board certification is through the National Certification Board for Therapeutic Massage and Bodywork and is required for licensing in at least 20 of the 29 states that regulate massage therapists.

Podiatrists

Podiatrists are foot care professionals who hold a doctor of podiatric medicine degree (DPM). They complete a bachelor's degree plus 4 years of medical training at one of the country's seven colleges of podiatric medicine. Many states require an additional 1-year residency of postdoctoral work before licensure. Some podiatrists are board certified in podiatric surgery.

Chiropractors

Chiropractic was developed in the United States in 1885. Doctors of chiropractic (DC) use adjustment and manipulation of the body, primarily the spine, to treat musculoskeletal disorders such as low back pain. They do not dispense prescription drugs (although many suggest specific herbals and supplements) or perform surgery. Chiropractors attend 4-year chiropractic colleges and are licensed by the state in which they practice. Certification is through the National Board of Chiropractic Examiners.

Acupuncturists

Acupuncture originated in ancient China and is used to control pain by the stimulation of "acupoints" by various methods. It is based on the theory that an essential life energy called "qi" flows through the body along invisible meridians. Stimulation of points along these meridians corrects the flow of qi to optimize health or block pain.

Acupuncturists can be certified by one of two methods. Educational training can include a formal, full-time educational program consisting of 1,725 hours or an apprenticeship program requiring 4,000 hours in a 3- to 6-year period. They must also have completed a "Clean Needle Technique" approved course. Medical doctors can complete 220 hours of training in acupuncture to be considered for board certification.

Certification for formally trained acupuncturists is through the National Certification Commission for Acupuncture and Oriental Medicine. Medical doctors are certified through the American Academy of Medical Acupuncture and must possess a valid medical license. As of January 2001, of the 40 states that regulate the profession of acupuncture, 37 states required certification for licensure.

Homeopaths

Homeopathy was developed in 18th century Germany and is based on the theory that "like cures like." Miniscule amounts of natural substances such as herbs, minerals, and animal products are used to provoke the body of a sick person to heal an illness through their administration in a serially diluted preparation. Three states (AZ, CT, NV) license homeopaths, and they require a DO or MD degree and a certificate in the study of homeopathy. While a board examination is offered, it is not required for licensure. Certification is offered through the Council for Homeopathic Certification. Five hundred training hours in classic homeopathy or 2,000 hours of an apprenticeship are required for membership in the Council.

Naturopaths

Naturopathy began in 19th century Europe, and its underlying principles revolve around encouraging healthy living habits and allowing the body to heal itself. Naturopathic physicians (NDs) have expertise in nutrition and frequently work in conjunction with physicians or other health care providers. They also can treat wounds and are trained in minor surgery. NDs complete a 4-year training program that includes nontoxic therapies such as homeopathy, clinical nutrition, manipulation, herbal medicine, and hydrotherapy. They often may have additional training in Chinese medicine (acupuncture and herbs). Naturopaths are licensed in 12 states. Certification is offered by the North American Board of Naturopathic Examiners.

GETTING THE MOST OUT OF YOUR DOCTOR VISIT

Ideally, a doctor-patient relationship is a partnership. But you have to hold up your end in order for your treatment to be as effective as possible. If you prepare for your doctor visit ahead of time, you won't come away with more questions than when you went in.

Try these tips for being an effective partner with your doctor and the rest of your health care team.

The First Visit

If you aren't familiar with the doctor's office, call to get directions and ask about parking. Leave early so you'll have plenty of time to find the office and park. That extra time will also be helpful once you arrive, since you'll need to fill out a form with basic information and your medical history before you see the doctor.

Before You Arrive

Jot down details of your medical history, even those that aren't related to the reason for your visit. Note any allergies you have and any medications you are taking. Take your insurance card or referral. Take any lab tests and X-rays or other imaging studies related to the condition. Be sure to inform your doctor about any over-the-counter medications, nutritional supplements, vitamins, or herbs you are taking. Also be sure to tell your doctor about other practitioners you may be seeing, such as a massage therapist, chiropractor, homeopath, or naturopath.

Wear comfortable clothes that you can remove easily for the examination.

Talking to the Doctor

Your appointment time will be limited, so make it as efficient as possible. Stick to the point and answer the doctor's questions directly and honestly. Don't hold back if you have concerns about subjects you might think are embarrassing such as incontinence or sexual problems. The doctor is there to help you (and has heard it all before). Ask for clarification if you don't understand what the doctor is saying. It's also a good idea to take notes because it's easy to forget parts of the conversation after you leave. Repeat instructions such as how and when to take medication if you aren't sure you heard correctly. If you are anxious about seeing the doctor and are worried that you won't remember everything, take along a family member to the appointment. You can also get additional information from the nurse, physical therapist, or others working with the doctor on your case.

After the Visit

If you can't figure out something in your notes or forgot to ask a question, call the doctor's office and ask for additional information.

Following the doctor's instructions will make the recommended treatment more effective. It's especially important that you take all the medication prescribed. If you have a 14-day course of pills, don't stop taking them on day 5 just because you feel better. If the doctor recommended a specific diet or exercise routine, stick to it. And keep your doctor informed if your condition changes or if there is no improvement.

If You Need Surgery

If your doctor recommends surgery, you'll probably have a lot of questions. Here are the most important things to find out:

1. Why is this procedure being recommended and what are the alternatives?

2. What are the benefits and how long will they last?

3. What are the risks of the procedure? How is it done?

4. What percentage of patients improves following this surgery?

5. What if I don't have the surgery now?

6. Do you perform this type of surgery or will I be referred to someone else? If it's someone else, ask if that doctor is board certified and if you can meet with him or her. Find out how many similar procedures this surgeon has done and what the outcomes were.

7. What kind of anesthesia will be used and what are the risks and possible after effects?

8. Will I have pain after the surgery?

9. How long will recovery take? Will I need help at home and, if so, for how long?

10. Will I have disability following the surgery and will I need physical therapy?

11. When will I be able to resume my normal activities including driving my car?

12. Whom can I consult for a second opinion?

13. Do I need to stop any medications, herbs, or supplements before surgery?

Insurance and Second Opinions

Before deciding on surgery, it's wise to ask your insurance company whether or to what extent the procedure will be covered and how the claim will be processed and paid.

Many insurers and managed care companies require clearance or precertification for surgery and/or second opinions. Find out what yours requires.

Writing It All Down

1. What should I expect from the recommended treatment?

2. How it will affect my daily activities?

3. How can I prevent the problem in the future?

4. Do you have any handouts describing my problem or its treatment?

5. Can you recommend a website or video program?

6. Would any alternative therapy be helpful or potentially harmful?

If the surgery involves more than just a minor procedure or if you are unsure about whether to go ahead with it, it's a good idea to get a second opinion even if your insurance company doesn't

require it. Doctors are used to this and won't be offended. You can ask for a referral either from your family physician or from your specialist.

MEDICATIONS

A number of medications, both over-the-counter and prescription, are used to treat musculoskeletal problems. Though manufacturers may claim that one drug is better than another, patients vary in their response to these medications. Therefore, if one does not provide you with pain relief, try another.

Most of these medications fall into two broad categories. Here's a short primer on the medicines your doctor may recommend.

NSAIDs

The broad category of nonsteroidal anti-inflammatory drugs includes medications that not only relieve pain but also reduce inflammation and swelling. Over-the-counter NSAIDs that you are probably familiar with include various brands of ibuprofen, naproxen, and aspirin. These drugs are sometimes called analgesics, which means pain relievers. An array of prescription

NSAIDs are also available if the over-the-counter medications fail to adequately relieve symptoms.

The main side effect of these medicines is stomach irritation. Also, people with ulcers, asthma, or kidney or liver disease may not be able to take NSAIDs safely.

An NSAID usually can be taken for a long period of time, if needed, and without your body building up resistance to the drug. However, most doctors recommend that if you take an NSAID longer than 6 months you should have blood tests to make sure the drug isn't causing liver or kidney damage or other side effects.

Corticosteroids

These drugs—such as prednisone, cortisone, and hydrocortisone—have an even greater ability to reduce inflammation than NSAIDs. These drugs can be administered through injections, orally, and in topical medications such as ointments or creams.

Talk To Your Doctor

Keep your doctor informed of the over-the-counter medications, dietary supplements, and herbs you are taking and also any other drugs that may have been prescribed for you by another doctor to treat an unrelated condition. Medications can interact with each other, causing one to be less effective or possibly causing dangerous interactions. Also, don't stop taking your medication without talking to your doctor. This is especially important if you are on corticosteroids, since stopping them suddenly, rather reducing your dose gradually, can be harmful.

Read the information that comes with your medications, follow the instructions for taking them, and call your doctor immediately if you experience unusual symptoms. Any unusual symptom might be a sign of an allergic reaction.

Although these drugs are stronger, they also can cause more serious side effects, especially with long-term use. Liquid cortisone, for example, can be injected directly into a joint to temporarily relieve pain, but doctors must limit how often they do this in the same joint because tissue damage can eventually occur.

Short-term side effects of oral corticosteroids include swelling, increased appetite, weight gain, and emotional highs and lows. The oral form is useful, however, in relieving acute pain from an inflammation caused by a herniated disk in the neck or back. This medication is also used for patients with rheumatoid arthritis (RA) when multiple joints are infected and injecting corticosteroids is not practical.

DMARDs

A third category of drug, disease-modifying anti-rheumatic drugs, is sometimes used to treat arthritis. These drugs not only relieve pain and inflammation but also can help control the progression of the disease. They may be tried when NSAIDs fail to ease symptoms, or they may be taken in combination with NSAIDs. Examples of DMARDs include methotrexate, sulfasalazine, and gold salt injections.

Understanding Imaging Techniques

Among a doctor's most valuable diagnostic tools are X-rays and other imaging techniques. These allow a view inside the body's tissues so the doctor can assess damage and determine treatment.

X-Rays

An X-ray, sometimes called a radiograph, is the most commonly used imaging method for musculoskeletal problems. It can show fractures, joint deformities, bone spurs, and other problems in hard tissue (bone) (see figures, left, below). The small amount of radiation used to expose the X-ray film is not harmful to you, but you should let your doctor know if you are pregnant so that extra precautions can be taken.

An X-ray itself is painless, but occasionally the procedure is uncomfortable if you have to hold your injured extremity in a particular position while the image is being taken. Fortunately, an X-ray only takes a few seconds. Often, the doctor will need to take more than one shot while you move the affected area into different positions to allow for views from different sides or angles. If one limb is fractured, the doctor may X-ray the uninjured side to get a comparison picture.

An X-ray is the least expensive and fastest of the imaging techniques and can be done in a doctor's office that has the necessary equipment and staff. Sometimes the doctor will combine X-rays with more sophisticated imaging procedures such as MRI or CT scans that can provide additional

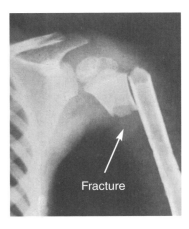
Fracture

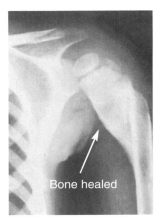
Bone healed

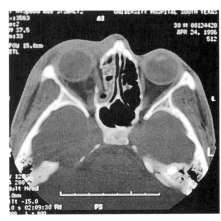

detail. X-rays are used not only for an initial diagnosis, but may be repeated following treatment to determine whether the bone has healed properly.

Computed Tomography (CT Scan)

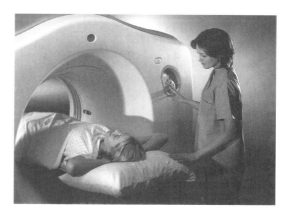

A CT scan takes fraction-of-a-second X-rays that pass through a body part at different angles and then can be combined in a computer image to provide a cross-sectional view (see figure, right, p 16). Doctors sometimes use it to view complex fractures in bones or joints when a simple X-ray can't provide as much detail. Although soft tissues will also be visible, they don't show up as well as the bones.

The procedure is painless. You lie very still on a table that is attached to a machine shaped somewhat like a fat donut. During the procedure, the table moves into the opening in the donut where an X-ray tube rotates around your body taking pictures from all directions. Because the equipment is very expensive, this technology is typically available only in hospitals or radiology facilities. Usually, a CT scan takes 30 to 40 minutes. To diagnose certain conditions, the doctor may inject a dye to make certain parts of the body show up better.

The Use and Effects of Dyes

Sometimes contrast material, often an iodine-based dye, is injected prior to an imaging test so that different body structures show up more clearly. You may feel hot when the dye is first injected and may also notice a metallic taste in your mouth, but these symptoms usually go away in a minute or two. Some people have minor allergic reactions to the dye such as itching, hives, or sneezing, but these can easily be treated. In rare cases, patients have more serious allergic reactions including difficulty breathing. If this happens during the test, tell the medical professional immediately so you can be given a counteracting medication. People allergic to shellfish are often sensitive to iodine. If you have reacted to iodine before, you might still be able to have the test by taking medications beforehand that can help minimize an allergic reaction.

Magnetic Resonance Imaging (MRI)

MRI, also painless, uses powerful magnet and radio waves to produce a series of cross-sectional images of a part of the body. It has the advantage of being able to show damage in soft tissues such as muscles, ligaments, tendons and cartilage (see figure below).

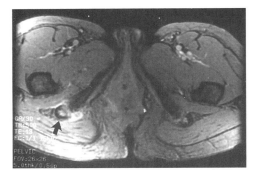

The more common type of scanner, a "closed" scanner, looks like a long tube, opened at both ends. You lie very still on a table inside the tube. An intercom allows you to communicate with the operator during the test. The equipment is noisy, so you'll be given headphones to muffle the banging

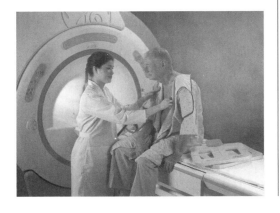

sounds. (If it's the lower part of your body that is being scanned, the upper part of your body doesn't need to be in the tube.)

You cannot wear anything metal into the scanner, so leave your jewelry or other metal items at home.

People who suffer from claustrophobia can request a sedative before undergoing the MRI.

Newer technology has spawned "open" MRI scanners that are smaller, donut-shaped devices that allow your head and most of your body to remain outside the magnet tube while one portion is scanned. Some doctors' offices now have these devices so you won't have to go to a hospital or radiology facility as would typically be the case with a closed MRI.

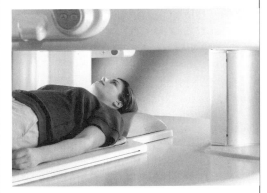

MRIs can take as little as 30 minutes or more than an hour. Sometimes during the procedure, you are given an intravenous (IV)

injection of dye that helps highlight normal and abnormal areas
in the body part being examined.

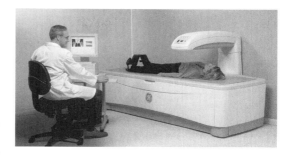

Arthrography

This is a less expensive technique
than MRI or CT scan and involves
the injection of contrasting dye
into a joint to highlight abnormalities on an X-ray. Arthrography is
useful in revealing some types of
ligament and cartilage tears. It
was used more frequently prior to
the advent of MRI and CT scan.
Sometimes arthrography is used
in combination with an MRI or CT
scan. Again, because dye is used
as contrast material, patients who
are allergic may have trouble with
this test.

Bone Scan

With this procedure (also called
bone scintigraphy), a small
amount of radioactive material is
injected into the bloodstream and
absorbed by the bone. Some
patients might feel a slight burning sensation or feeling of being
flushed or warm as the material
is injected, while others say it
feels no different than a regular
injection. Between 3 and 6 hours
after the injection, the patient is
placed in a scanner that detects
the amount of the material that
has been absorbed in the bones.
By showing blood flow and metabolic activity within the bone, the
test can reveal abnormalities
such as bone damage. The
radioactive material is picked up
by the area of the bone that is
trying to repair itself, such as in a
stress fracture. When this happens, doctors say the scan "lights
up" or is "hot."

THE "HEALTHY BONES" DIET

When you were a child, you probably heard that "drinking milk
builds strong bones." But did you
know that this message is just as
important when your bone density peaks at around age 35? Your
need for calcium continues
throughout life. Even if you aren't
a milk drinker, you can get this
important mineral from other
sources. Trouble is, most of us
don't eat enough calcium-rich
foods to reach our minimum daily
requirements.

Bone is a living tissue that is constantly remodeling, a process in which small amounts of old bone cells are shed and replaced with new cells. After 35, you lose more than you gain, and the loss accelerates for women after menopause. (See p 48 for information on osteoporosis.) Since your body doesn't make calcium, you need to get it through the foods you eat, starting in childhood.

Doctors like to describe the process as a "bone bank." If you deposit plenty of calcium when you are younger, your bones will be stronger when you get older. Milk, cheese, yogurt, and other dairy products are an excellent source. So are green vegetables such as kale and broccoli. You can also eat foods that are fortified with calcium, including some cereals, breakfast bars, and orange juice. And you can add 2 to 4 tablespoons of nonfat powdered milk to puddings, custards, hot cereals, and baked goods for a calcium boost.

Calcium-Rich Foods

Serving Size	Food	Amount of Calcium (mg)
1 cup (8 oz)	Yogurt (plain low fat)	415
1 cup	Yogurt (fruit low fat)	314
1 cup	Skim milk	302
1 cup	2% milk	297
1 oz	Swiss cheese	272
1 oz	Cheddar cheese	204
1 oz	Colby cheese	194
1 oz	Cottage cheese, low fat	155
10 fl oz	Vanilla shake	344
1 cup	Vanilla ice cream	170
1 cup	Tofu	260
1½ cup	Chef salad	235
1 cup	Almonds	332
1 cup, chopped	Collard greens, cooked	357
1 cup, chopped	Kale, cooked	179
1 cup	Broccoli, cooked	94

Vitamin D

Vitamin D plays a crucial role in bone health, too, because it is necessary for calcium to be absorbed. Vitamin D is made by the skin following exposure to sunlight. The National Osteoporosis Foundation reports that 10 to 15 minutes of exposure of the hands, arms, and face two or three times a week is generally enough to fit the body's requirements.

You can also get vitamin D through fortified dairy products, egg yolks, saltwater fish, and liver. It's found in most multivitamins and in some calcium supplements.

People with limited sun exposure need to get vitamin D through their diet. The recommended daily intake is 400 to 600 IU (international units). You can get 400 IU from four 8-oz glasses of skim milk, for example.

What About Supplements?

Many people find it difficult to consume enough calcium through diet alone. Some individuals are lactose intolerant, meaning that they have trouble digesting dairy foods. Others worry about eating foods high in fat, such as cheese, or they just don't like drinking milk. That's why calcium supplements are popular.

How Much is Enough?

The National Academy of Sciences' Institute of Medicine offers these guidelines for daily calcium intake.

1. *800 mg for children 4 to 8 years*
2. *1,300 mg for children 9 to 18 years*
3. *1,000 mg for men and women 19 to 50 years (including pregnant or nursing women)*
4. *1,300 mg for pregnant or nursing women under age 18*
5. *1,200 mg for men and women over 50 years*

Strive for reaching the recommendations, but don't overdo it. People who regularly consume more than 2,500 mg a day are at risk for kidney problems.

Supplements come in several forms. You can swallow a pill or chew a tablet, drink a liquid or eat a chewy candy-type supplement. Whatever you choose, check the label to make sure the supplement you buy meets *US Pharmacopeia* (USP) standards. Take the supplement just before or during a meal, and take only 500 mg at a time.

Check with your doctor before taking calcium supplements because they can cause interactions with other drugs you may be taking such as iron supplements or tetracycline, an antibiotic.

THE POWERS OF EXERCISE

Throughout *The 2003 Body Almanac* you've read repeatedly that the way to prevent myriad problems of bones and muscles is through exercise. You don't have to be a marathon runner to get the benefits. Moderate activity, if done regularly, can affect how you feel now and how mobile you will remain into old age.

Even if you are already physically active, you may not be maximizing your exercise time. Maybe yours is strictly an aerobics workout, which is good for your cardiovascular system but doesn't do much for your muscle strength. Or maybe you are risking injury because you push your body too hard or because you aren't using the proper technique. These are

The Weight Connection

There's another reason why diet is important to healthy bones. Being overweight puts extra strain on bones and joints and can lead to overuse injuries in areas such as the knees and hips. Here are tips for keeping the weight off.

1. *Get some weight-bearing exercise, which not only trims fat but strengthens bones. Try brisk walking, jogging, hiking, dancing, weight training.*

2. *Get your kids moving, too. Enroll them in sports activities that involve running, take them to the playground, go on a nature walk, or take a hike.*

3. *Limit your family's TV watching. It promotes snacking and keeps you from moving.*

4. *Limit soft drink consumption and choose milk instead.*

5. *Limit your family's trips to fast food restaurants.*

6. *Keep healthy snacks in your refrigerator so kids (and adults!) can easily help themselves.*

7. *If you think your child is becoming overweight, talk to your pediatrician or a nutritionist who specializes in helping kids make better food choices.*

common mistakes exercisers make. Read on for tips on how to get the most from your workout and do it safely.

General Guidelines

1. Check with your doctor before beginning a new exercise regimen if you have a chronic condition such as arthritis, diabetes, a cardiovascular condition or past orthopaedic injuries, or if you are a smoker, overweight or middle-aged or older and haven't exercised before. Choose something you enjoy so you'll be more likely to stick with it. Consider different activities on different days so you don't get bored with your workout.

2. Start gradually and build up the intensity and length of your workout. If you plunge in with a strenuous program, you may lose motivation and also risk being injured.

3. Buy the right kind of shoes; especially if you are jogging, and check them periodically for wear. Runners who log up to 10 miles a week, for example, should replace their shoes every 9 to 12 months to maintain adequate levels of shock absorption. (See p 234 for buying advice.)

4. Set a weekly schedule for exercise that includes some days off. You might start with workouts every other day.

5. Keep a water bottle handy during your workout to avoid dehydration, especially if you are exercising outside in warm temperatures. Cold muscles are more prone to injury. At the beginning of your exercise routine, do a few minutes of stretching exercises. After your workout, spend 5 minutes cooling your muscles down again with gentle stretches.

6. Don't stop exercising if your muscles become sore in the beginning. The soreness will go away as you continue to exercise. But stop exercising if you experience severe pain or swelling as this could signal an injury.

7. Learn the proper technique for whatever exercise program you undertake. Even an activity as simple as brisk walking can yield better results if performed a certain way. Look for books or articles on your particular activity or seek the advice of a fitness trainer.

FIT is It!

To reap the benefits of aerobic exercise, remember FIT: Frequency, Intensity and Time.

Frequency: *Exercise at least three times a week.*

Intensity: *Work at an intensity level that reaches 60% to 80% of your maximum heart rate. This is called your target heart rate. You calculate it by subtracting your age from 220 and then figuring 60% to 80% of that. For example, if you are 50, your maximum rate is 170 and your target heart rate is in the range of 102 to 136. To determine whether you've reached your target, take your pulse immediately after you stop exercising, count the beats for 15 seconds, and multiply by four.*

Time: *Exercise at least 20 minutes during each session. If you are just beginning your exercise program, start with just 5 minutes and gradually work up from there. Your routine should always include an additional 5 minutes of warm-up stretching at the beginning and 5 minutes of cooldown at the end.*

Balancing Your Workout

For a total body workout, you need three types of activity in your routine—aerobic, strength training, and flexibility exercises. Balancing your routine by cross training also keeps you motivated!

Aerobic Exercise

Aerobic activity, such as brisk walking, running, swimming, dancing, or biking, strengthen your heart and lungs—cardiovascular system—through continuous, rhythmic activity of the large muscles in the legs and buttocks.

Strength Training

Strength training, such as weight lifting and push-ups, helps keep muscles and bones strong. This becomes especially important as we age and bone mass starts to decline. Weight training can be used for other purposes too, such as building up a specific muscle group for improved sports performance or to rehabilitate an injured muscle. If you are already doing aerobic exercise, you can incorporate strength training into your routine just twice a week and reap benefits. If you are focusing on a specific muscle group for sports, perform weight training only every other day so the muscles have time to recover.

Weight training adds resistance to body movements so that the moves are more difficult and the muscles adapt by working harder and becoming stronger. You can use free weights or a weight machine, either in a gym or in your home. Free weights are less expensive and adapt easily to smaller or larger body types. Weight machines are safer because the weight is more controlled.

A weight-training program should be designed around your physical condition and your reason for doing it—building muscles as opposed to rehabilitation, for example. If you want help in creating a program that's right for you, consult an exercise professional. If you are over 30 or have any physical limitations, check with your doctor before beginning any weight-training program.

Stretching Exercises

We've already mentioned the importance of stretching to warm up your muscles before a workout. Stretching improves your flexibility by keeping your muscles limber and helps prevent injury. A sample flexibility program appears on pp 65-70.

For some people, stretching is not just a quick warm up but a whole exercise routine. Yoga and Pilates are examples of popular stretching routines that also build strength and endurance. There

are several types of yoga, but they all use a combination of breathing exercises, stretching, and assuming various postures in order to reduce stress and improve flexibility and fitness. Pilates was originally designed for dancers and combines stretching and strengthening in fluid-like movements. Both yoga and Pilates are done on mats, although some Pilates workouts in gyms also incorporate special equipment.

Preventing Sports Injuries

Do you play sports to keep active? You'll be able to stay in the game if you follow some simple steps for avoiding injuries.

Sports injuries are classified as either "acute" or caused by "overuse."

Putting It All Together

With cross training, you incorporate all three elements. For example, your program could look something like this.

1. *Three times a week: 30 minutes of aerobics.*

2. *Twice a week on non-consecutive days: 30 minutes of weight training working each major muscle group.*

3. *Every day: 5 to 10 minutes of stretching.*

An acute injury is one in which a sudden event—a fall or a collision with another player, for example—causes damage such as a broken bone, torn cartilage, strained muscle, or sprained ligament.

An overuse injury is caused by repeated stress on a particular part of the body, eventually resulting in damage. Examples include tendinitis and stress fractures.

Specific injuries are described throughout this book. The tips that follow will help you play safer.

Playing Safe

Warm up. Cold muscles are more vulnerable to injury. Do some stretching and warm-up exercises (such jumping jacks or running in place) before plunging into an intense level of activity.

Don't be a "weekend warrior." If you don't do anything all week and then play hard on the weekend, you can put too much stress on your bones and muscles. It won't really improve your fitness level, either. Try to get in 30 minutes of moderate activity every day, even if you have to break it into 10-minute blocks. Take the stairs instead of the elevator, take a walk on your lunch hour, or run around the block with your dog, for example.

Average Calories Burned* from One Hour of Activity	
Walking the dog	250
Walking briskly	281
Climbing stairs	563
Gardening	352
Mowing the lawn	387
Pushing baby in stroller	176
Housecleaning	246
* Based on person weighing 155 lb	

Take lessons. If you are new to the sport or even if you've played for a while, you can benefit from instruction that ensures you use proper form, thereby reducing the risk of an overuse injury.

Use proper equipment. A tennis racket with a grip that fits your hand, for example, will put less stress on your hand and arm than a grip that doesn't. If you take up in-line skating, wear all the recommended protective equipment including knee and wrist pads and a helmet.

Use equipment properly. A bike helmet, for example, doesn't provide as much protection if it's not positioned over the forehead, yet this is a common mistake among bike riders.

Wear the right shoes. Lots of injuries could be prevented if athletes were more careful about the shoes they wear for sports. (See p 234 for how to buy the right pair.)

Don't go too far too fast. Even if you have been playing a sport for a while, don't increase your activity level suddenly. Increase your playing time gradually to prevent overuse injuries.

Listen to your body. If you play through pain, you can turn a minor injury into a major one. And if you suffer an injury, follow your doctor's advice about how long to lay off your sport and how to get back in shape before resuming. This helps you avoid re-injuring yourself.

GETTING KIDS READY FOR SPORTS

More kids than ever are playing sports. The number of children participating in both formal and informal sports is growing, especially among girls. This is good news since children who are physically active are building strong bones and muscles. They also become more self-confident and improve both their agility and coordination. And, if they develop the habit of physical activity in childhood, it's more likely that they will grow up to be physically active adults.

Minor bumps, scrapes, and bruises are an inevitable part of the game. The benefits of an active lifestyle—and the fun of playing—are worth that small price. But serious injuries are another matter—parents and coaches can do a lot to prevent them. Here are some ways to keep your young athlete in the game.

Warm Up

Cold muscles are more prone to injury. Teach your kids to warm up their muscles with 5 to 10 minutes of the same types of stretching exercises that adults do before beginning a practice or a game. Focus especially on the calf and thigh muscles. After playing, they should spend 5 minutes cooling their muscles down again with gentle stretches or just walking around for a few minutes.

Keep Them Fed and Watered

Give your children water bottles to take to practices and remind them to take frequent water breaks so they stay hydrated in hot weather. Provide a sports (dilute glucose-electrolyte) drink instead of just water if the activity will last longer than an hour and is intense enough to produce a lot of sweating. One benefit of fluid replacement drinks is that kids tend to prefer them to plain water, so they'll consume more. A snack before practice such as a banana or peanut butter on a bagel helps keep them fueled.

Wear Protective Gear

Many sports call for a helmet, padding, shoes with cleats or other safety equipment. Require your kids to wear this gear for both practices and games. Check periodically to make sure the equipment still fits your growing children and that they are wearing the gear properly according to the manufacturer's directions.

Buy the Right Shoes

The right athletic shoes with the right fit can do a lot to prevent leg and foot injuries ranging from blisters to tendinitis. (See p 234 for tips on buying the right shoes.)

Avoid Overdoing It

Some kids play too long and too hard, resulting in overuse injuries. Concern about this led the Little League and other national youth baseball organizations, for example, to establish rules that limit the number of

innings an individual player may pitch, depending on age. (See p 97 for recommendations.) Some children play on more than one team per season or play more than one sport simultaneously; parents must guard against children overworking their bodies in these situations. Also, teach your children to read their body's signals. They should not play through pain or when they become overly tired.

Follow the Rules

Many sports rules are written specifically to prevent injuries. Make sure all team members know the rules and follow them.

Don't Overemphasize Competition

Too much stress on winning can lead to injuries. Let kids play for the fun of it. Some will develop a competitive spirit on their own, and that's okay. But it shouldn't be pushed on them by overzealous adults; disastrous results can ensue. An example of this is when parents pressure their kids to play competitively at very young ages.

Kids Should Be Grouped by Size and Skill

Using chronologic age to decide on team assignments, especially in contact sports, can lead to injuries because this system

The Coach's Job

Many youth sports leagues rely on parent volunteers to serve as coaches. The best ones take advantage of training opportunities so they not only learn how to teach the fundamentals of the game but also how to prevent injuries. Ideally, coaches will have had first aid and CPR training. There should be a fully stocked first aid kit handy at all practices and games and a cell phone so the coach can summon help in an emergency.

mixes kids of different physical maturity. A 15-year-old who is 180 lb and 6' tall is a dangerous match-up for a competitor of the same age who weighs only 135 lb and 5' 3" tall. If age must be

used, the coaches should try to modify the game to accommodate kids of different sizes.

As for gender differences, coed teams are fine until youngsters reach puberty. At that point, same-sex teams are safer because boys gain muscle mass and tend to be bigger and stronger than most girls. Exceptions can be made for an outstanding female player for whom there is no girls' team.

Get a Physical

Take your child for a medical exam before he or she starts a competitive sport. Many athletes use ergogenic aids, which are substances that reportedly enhance performance. Many of these substances are dangerous; some are potentially fatal. You must discuss the use of these with your doctor.

IS IT BROKEN?

What It Is

At some point in your life, you've probably had an injury and wondered whether you might have broken a bone. Or maybe this has happened to your child. Is it just a simple sprain you can treat yourself? How can you decide?

Signs and Symptoms

Some fractures are obvious—if the bone is so badly broken that a portion is sticking out from the skin or the injured body part looks deformed. You may even hear the bone crack. But often, the signs aren't so obvious, and the only

Two Types Of Fractures

Closed or simple fracture

The bone is broken but it hasn't pierced the skin. Immobilize the injured area with a splint (and a sling in the case of an arm or shoulder injury) to keep the area more comfortable while you head to a doctor or hospital emergency room.

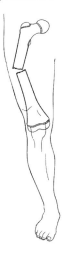

Open or compound fracture

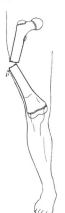

There is an open wound. This can either be because the broken end of the bone pierced the skin or because the blow that caused the break also caused a wound. In this type of fracture, apply pressure with a clean cloth to stop bleeding and then summon medical help immediately.

way to know for sure is to have the bone X-rayed. The question is whether you need to head for the hospital emergency room. Just because you can move the injured body part—such as a hand or foot—doesn't mean it isn't broken.

A possible broken bone can be even harder to judge in children because they might cry long and loud from falls, whether anything is broken or not. Fear alone can make children cry. And young ones may not be able to communicate how much pain they are in or exactly where the pain is greatest. Older children, especially those playing sports, may be stoic after an injury to avoid embarrassment in front of teammates, even though they are in a lot of pain.

Broken bones are more common in children than adults because their smaller bones break more easily and because they are more active. Kids' broken bones also heal more quickly than those of adults. Most of the injuries occur because of falls.

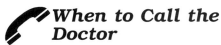

When to Call the Doctor

A broken bone will be very painful and cause swelling. These can be signs of sprains, too, but if your child refuses to use the limb for longer than 30 minutes because of the pain, a fracture is a strong possibility and needs prompt medical attention for a proper diagnosis.

The risk of fractures in adults increases with age since bones weaken due to osteoporosis. If you sustain an injury, even a minor one, and can't use that part of your body within 30 minutes because of pain and swelling, assume that it might not be just a sprain and seek medical attention. Untreated fractures mistaken for sprains can heal improperly and may cause traumatic arthritis or other problems later.

If the broken bone breaks the skin, call 9-1-1 immediately.

How to Treat It

The injury will be X-rayed and, if a fracture is confirmed, the injury will be immobilized in a cast or splint. In some cases, surgery is necessary to realign the bone so it can heal.

Prevention

Keeping bones strong through adequate calcium intake and weight-bearing exercise can help. See individual chapters for more ideas on protecting specific body parts.

CARE OF CASTS AND SPLINTS

Although it may seem like a nuisance to have to wear a cast or splint when you break a bone, just remember that it's speeding the healing process while giving you the freedom to continue many of your regular activities. A fracture cannot heal if there is motion at the site where the break has occurred. By holding the two parts of the bone together, the cast or splint allows bone tissue to fill in the crack. You'll need to do your part by taking care of your cast or splint.

A cast is custom-made by your health care professional, either with plaster or fiberglass material in strips or rolls that become flexible when dipped in water. The skin over the injured area is first covered with cotton or synthetic padding then wrapped with the wet cast material that quickly hardens as it dries.

Plaster casts are less expensive than fiberglass and in some cases can be shaped better to fit an injury.

Comparing Casts and Splints

	Construction	Advantages
Plaster Cast	Custom-made	Less expensive than fiberglass Can be shaped better to fit injury
Fiberglass Cast	Custom-made	Lighter weight than plaster Breathes better Wears longer
Splint (half cast)	Custom-made or off the shelf	Accommodates swelling better than closed cast Easy to remove with Velcro straps

Fiberglass casts weigh less, wear longer, and breath better than plaster. An X-ray to check the progress of healing can see through fiberglass more easily than through plaster.

A splint, or half cast, provides less support because it doesn't completely surround the limb. The advantage is that a splint can be more easily adjusted to accommodate swelling than can a closed cast. Splints can be custom made when an exact fit is necessary, but sometimes an off-the-shelf model works fine too. These have Velcro straps for easy removal and adjustment.

Sometimes a splint is applied first until the swelling goes down and then a full cast is applied. Your doctor will decide which type of support is best for your specific injury.

Coping with Casts and Splints the First Few Days

Here are some general guidelines for dealing with your cast or splint, but ask your doctor for specific instructions.

Swelling can cause a cast to feel tight in the first 48 to 72 hours. Reducing early swelling will ease the pain and speed the healing process.

To reduce swelling, elevate the injured limb above your heart to keep the blood flowing downhill. For example, prop up a broken arm or leg on pillows. Also, put ice in a dry plastic bag or ice pack and loosely wrap it around the splint or cast at the site of the injury. Move uninjured but swollen fingers and toes gently and often.

Caring for Your Splint or Cast

Caring for your cast or splint is sometimes very trying. It's important, however, so that the cast can continue to do its job. A wet or damaged cast or splint will not provide the immobilization your bones or joint needs. The result can be delayed healing (called nonunion) or improper healing (called malunion). In either case, your treatment will be longer, or worse, you may have problems with pain and resulting deformity.

Therefore, you should follow these simple guidelines to make sure that your cast can do its job.

1. Keep it dry. To shower or bathe, use two layers of plastic or buy waterproof shields.

2. Don't pull out the padding.

3. Don't stick objects such as coat hangers inside to scratch itchy skin.

4. Keep dirt, sand, and powder away from the inside of the cast. If itching persists or if

Signs of Trouble

Call your doctor immediately if you notice any of these symptoms, which could indicate the cast is causing too much pressure:

1. *increased pain and a feeling that the cast is too tight*

2. *numbness or tingling in the hand or foot*

3. *burning or stinging from too much pressure on the skin*

4. *excessive swelling below the cast from too little blood circulation*

5. *lost of active movement of toes or fingers*

the skin around the cast becomes irritated, call your doctor for advice.

5. Don't break off or trim rough edges of the cast without asking your doctor first. Let your doctor know if the cast becomes cracked or develops soft spots.

6. If you have a walking cast, don't walk on it until it hardens completely. This takes about 1 hour for fiberglass but 2 or 3 days for plaster casts.

TREATING WOUNDS

What It Is

? A wound is any cut or puncture of the skin. No matter how minor it seems, every wound needs prompt treatment to prevent infection. When the skin is broken because of a fracture, special handling is required. Here's a quick review on how to treat various types of wounds.

Cuts

If it's bleeding, cover the wound with a clean cloth and apply direct, continuous pressure with your hand. Usually, minor bleeding will slow or stop within about 10 minutes. Wash minor cuts thoroughly with soap and water, apply an antibiotic ointment, and cover the wound with a clean bandage. It's a good idea to take the bandage off a couple of times a day to let the wound breathe. Afterwards, apply a clean bandage to keep the wound clean but leave it off whenever possible, such as when you are sleeping, since exposure to air promotes healing.

Keep watch for signs of infection such as increased pain and swelling, warmth, red streaks, or pus draining. Infected wounds need prompt treatment by a medical professional.

If the bleeding is more serious, try elevating the wound higher than your heart to help stop the flow. Don't do this, however, if it causes more pain. If the bleeding doesn't slow after 15 minutes of direct pressure or if it is spurting out of the wound, call for medical help. However, don't ever apply a tourniquet because this can cause nerve and tissue damage.

Shock

Excessive bleeding can sometimes lead to shock, a condition that develops when there is reduced circulation of oxygen (via the blood) to the body's organs. Call 9-1-1 immediately if you notice any of the following symptoms with severe bleeding.

- Lightheadedness or weakness
- Shallow or rapid breathing,
- Thirst
- Nausea or vomiting
- Confusion
- Moist, cool skin or profuse sweating

Stitches

A cut that is long, deep, or has a gaping appearance or that bleeds a lot will probably need stitches. Prompt treatment by a doctor is especially important if the cut has damaged a nerve, a muscle, or tendon. If you aren't sure whether the cut needs stitches, especially if it's on your face or on an area that moves a lot such as the hand or the knee, have a doctor check it. Facial cuts can leave scars if not treated properly. Cuts on hands and knees can be slow to heal because the constant movement prevents the wound from staying closed.

Open Fractures

If a bone is sticking out of the wound, don't try to push it back. Cover the wound with a clean, dry dressing and call 9-1-1 immediately.

Puncture Wounds

Puncture wounds are particularly risky because they penetrate the tissue and deposit bacteria, which can then flourish in warm, moist conditions. Bites from humans or animals are especially prone to infection. (See below for more information.)

If you receive a minor puncture wound, such as from a pin, staple, or thumbtack, soak the wound in warm water for 20 minutes two to four times a day for 4 or 5 days. Exposure to air promotes healing, but bandage the wound if it's in a place that is likely to get dirty. With any cuts or puncture wounds, you should check to make sure your tetanus shot is up to date. Watch for the signs of infection listed below.

If the puncture wound is larger or deeper, such as from a stick or a nail, or from an animal or human bite, see your doctor as soon as possible as you may need to take antibiotics due to the high likelihood of infection.

Signs of Infection

Keep an eye on your wound as it heals. If you notice redness, swelling, warmth, increased pain, or fever, these are signs of infection and require immediate treatment by a doctor.

BITES

What It Is

? Animal and human bite wounds are common. The immediate concern is potential infection. If the bite is severe, there also can be direct damage

to tendons, muscles, nerves, or even bones. But infection is the biggest immediate concern.

Sometimes people delay seeking medical attention because the wound seems small. This is a

Who Bites Most Often?

They may be man's best friend, but dog bites account for 90% of animal bites. Cats are the second most common but only account for 5% of animal bites.

mistake because infection from human or animal bites can progress rapidly, and if untreated or if treatment is delayed, serious complications can develop.

You may have heard that dogs' mouths are cleaner than those of humans. It's true.

Although dog bite wounds can cause greater mechanical damage, the risk of infection from a cat bite is much higher—30% to 50%—than a dog bite because a cat's thin, sharp teeth can cause a deeper puncture wound. The various bacteria commonly found in cats' mouths differ from those in a dog's mouth and its germs are delivered well below the skin so washing the wound can't easily clean it. Thus the germs can easily multiply into an infection.

Signs and Symptoms

The skin is either punctured or cut, or there is an irregular, jagged wound. Naturally, the spot is painful. There may be little or no bleeding;

bleeding may indicate possible blood vessel damage. Swelling and redness may follow, which indicates the wound has become infected. If the bite is severe enough to cause loss of sensation or limited and painful motion, it's possible a tendon or nerve has been severed.

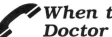

When to Call the Doctor

If the skin has been punctured, not just scratched superficially, call your doctor. If the skin is clearly punctured and the bite is from a cat or a human, you should see a doctor immediately. If the wound is ragged and bleeding, see a doctor.

When in doubt, call your doctor.

How to Treat It

Wash the wound immediately and thoroughly with soap and water. Apply a clean or sterile dressing and apply pressure to control any bleeding. Treatment most often includes a course of antibiotics since the risk of infection from bite wounds is so high. The type of antibiotic will depend on what type of bite has occurred. Wounds will need cleansing, and sometimes surgery to remove contamination or damaged tissue. Usually bite wounds are not stitched or sutured. Contrary to popular opinion, sutured wounds have a higher

What is the Risk of Rabies?

If the animal is unknown to you and you can't determine that it has an up-to-date rabies vaccination, report the incident to the local animal control authority. If the animal cannot be captured and confined for 10 days of observation to determine if it is healthy, you may need anti-rabies shots.

More than 90% of rabies in the United States comes from wild animals rather than pets. Bats, skunks, raccoons, and foxes are the most common carriers.

risk of infection than wounds left open to allow drainage of fluids. At times, wounds are sutured some days later when the risk of infection is lower.

Prevention

Teach your kids to treat pets gently. Children should not chase or tease animals or pull their tails. The Humane Society of the United States offers these additional tips.

1. If you don't know the dog (or cat), ask permission of the owner before trying to pet it. Then let the dog sniff your hand first before you touch it.

2. If a dog approaches you, stand still with your hands at your sides and don't make eye contact. Otherwise, you could appear threatening.

3. Don't run. A dog's instinct is to chase and catch you, but if you stand still, he'll likely just sniff you and then lose interest.

4. Don't pet a dog or cat while it's eating, sleeping, chewing a toy, or guarding something.

5. Don't approach an injured animal. Tell your children to tell an adult if they find one.

6. When you take your children to areas with wildlife, teach them not to approach wild animals to pet them or offer food. Not only does the child risk being bitten, but also "people" food can harm animals' digestive systems.

PREVENTING FALLS

Many fewer Americans would suffer injuries if they took simple precautions to prevent falls. They are the leading cause of injuries to people 65 and older. Your risk of falling could be cut in half by following simple safety measures. Although some of these tips apply more to the elderly, most of them are good common sense for people of any age, including children.

What to Wear

Wearing the wrong type of footwear can contribute to falls. Never walk around in stocking feet. Replace your slippers if they are loose or stretched out of shape. Avoid shoes with smooth, slick soles or soles that are extra thick. If you can't part with a favorite pair that has a slick sole, ask a shoe repair shop to added textured strips. Shoes with laces are safer than slip-ons, and the higher the heel, the greater the risk of falling, whether you are a teenager or a senior citizen.

Remember that clothes that are too long, such as coats, trousers, or bathrobes can trip you up.

Health Considerations

You may not realize that regular physicals can help prevent falls. Your health care provider may discover problems that can lead to dizziness, for example. Your doctor can also monitor side effects from your prescriptions and over-the-counter medications that might affect your balance.

Don't skip meals, especially not breakfast, because lack of food can make you feel dizzy. Maintain a diet with adequate calcium and vitamin D throughout your life to reduce the risk of a broken bone if you do fall.

Have an annual eye exam and wear glasses if you need them. But don't wear your reading glasses while walking around.

People of all ages can reduce their risk of falls through regular exercise. Even moderate physical activity can help you maintain your strength, coordination, agility, and balance.

Falling for Fido

Pets who sprawl on the floor can trip you. Since getting rid of pets just to prevent falls isn't something most people would consider, this points out the wisdom of walking only into well-lighted rooms and keeping an eye out for unexpected obstacles in your path.

Home Safety Checklist

1. Get rid of clutter. Don't pile newspapers on the floor, boxes on the stairway, or furnishings—plant stands, footstools, magazine racks, etc.—in pathways between rooms.

2. Keep appliance, lamp, and telephone cords out of areas where you walk. Don't put them under rugs, however, as the constant walking over the top can fray the cord and create a fire hazard.

3. Area rugs should be anchored with double-stick tape or slip-resist-ant backing. Get rid of small scatter rugs except in the bathroom, where a slip-resistant rug on a tile floor can make it easier to get in and out of the tub. Steps that are bare wood need nonslip treads. If you prefer carpeting on your stairs, avoid patterned, dark or deep pile carpeting. A solid, lighter color will show the step edges more clearly. If you have concrete, ceramic, or marble floors, car-peting not only reduces your risk of slipping but also cushions you if you do fall.

4. Good lighting is important. Light switches that are accessible when you enter a room prevent you from having to navigate a dark area to find a lamp. Glow-in-the-dark switches are an extra help. Make sure you have light switches at both the top and bottom of your stairways. Install a night-light along the route between your bed-room and bathroom. Consider adding motion detector lights, which turn on automatically, to your stairways and halls. Keep a flash-light by your bed in case of a power outage.

5. In the kitchen, clean up spills immediately. Don't stand on chairs or boxes to reach upper cabinets. Use a step stool or low steplad-der designed for this purpose, or better still, store things only where you can reach them easily. Also, use nonskid wax on your floor.

6. In the bathroom, use a rubber mat or put adhesive texture strips on the bottom of your tub. Seniors may feel safer with grab bars on the walls and a plastic seat in the tub along with a hand-held shower.

Playground Safety Checklist

1. Surfaces around equipment should have at least 12" of wood chips, mulch, sand or pea gravel, or rubber-like safety mats.

2. The protective surface should extend at least 6' in all directions from the piece of play equipment. For swings, the surface should extend, in back and front, twice the height of the suspending bar.

3. Play structures more than 30" high should be spaced at least 9' apart. Swings should be spaced far enough from each other and from the supporting posts to prevent impact.

4. Platforms, ramps, and other elevated surfaces should have guardrails to prevent falls.

5. Spaces that could trap children's heads, such as openings in guardrails or between ladder rungs should either be less than 3.5" or more than 9".

6. Check the playgrounds your children use to make sure the equipment is well maintained. Look especially for dangerous hardware such as open "S" hooks or protruding bolt ends that can catch on clothing and cause strangulation.

For more details on safe public playground or backyard equipment, contact the Consumer Products Safety Commission, www.cpsc.org or 1-800-638-2772.

Preventing Falls in Children

If you have a toddler in your home, install baby gates at the top and bottom of stairways. Install window guards on windows above the first floor. If you put them on windows that are also designated as possible exits in case of a fire, use guards that have quick release devices that only adults can open. Balconies, railings, and porches with railing spaces wider than 3" should be covered with plastic or mesh shields.

Grocery carts are another major cause of falls in children. Always use a safety strap when your child sits in the cart's seat, and don't let your child sit or stand in the basket where the food goes because this makes the cart top heavy.

Ladder Safety Checklist

Approximately half a million people a year are treated for injuries from falling off a ladder. Here's how to avoid becoming one of them.

1. Use a ladder that's the right height for the job. Inside the house, you probably need a low stepladder, but for outside jobs you may need a taller stepladder or an extension ladder. Ladders are also sized according to the working loads they can accommodate. The load includes the weight of the climber as well as the load being carried. Household ladders, for example, may only be designed to handle 200 lb, whereas an industrial-strength ladder may accommodate up to 300 lb.

2. Inspect your ladder and don't use it if it's damaged. Don't be tempted to make a temporary repair, as this could fail while you are on the ladder.

3. Place an extension ladder on firm, even ground with the bottom positioned 1' away from the wall for every 4' the ladder rises. If you are going all the way to your roof, the ladder should reach 3' higher than the roofline. Don't use a ladder in high winds.

4. A stepladder should be opened all the way and locked into position before you climb it.

5. Never stand on the top rung of a ladder and don't lean over the side or overreach. Instead, get down and move the ladder to a new location. And wear shoes with slip-resistant soles.

USING CANES, CRUTCHES, AND WALKERS

You may not relish having to use a walking aid, but it can make the difference between being stuck in a chair or getting on with your life when you have an injury or disability. You'll have more success if the aid you use is sized properly and you use it correctly. Here are some tips.

Canes

A cane is useful when you have a minor injury or a small problem with balance. But if it's too long or too short, a cane will put excess stress on your elbow and arm muscles. The top of the cane should reach the crease in your wrist when you stand up straight. Your elbow should be bent a little when you use it. If the weakness is on your left side, hold the cane in your right hand.

When you walk, swing your weak leg and the cane forward at the same time. If you are going up stairs, step up on your "good" leg first, grasping the cane in one hand and the railing—if there is one—with the other. Then step up on the injured leg. To descend, put the cane on the step first, then the injured leg and finally, your good leg.

Crutches

Any injury that requires you to keep weight off your leg or foot may put you on crutches for a while. The top of the crutches should be 1" to 1½" below your armpits when you stand up straight. The idea is for your hands to absorb the weight, not your armpits. The handgrips should be even with the top of your hip. At this setting, your elbows should bend a little when your hands are on the grips. Hold the crutches close to your body, lean forward slightly, put the crutches about a foot in front of

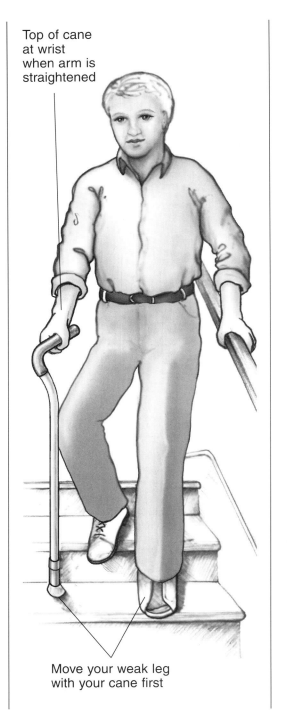

Top of cane at wrist when arm is straightened

Move your weak leg with your cane first

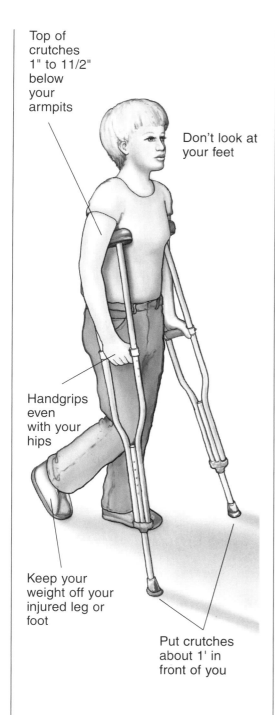

Top of
crutches
1" to 11/2"
below
your
armpits

Don't look at
your feet

Handgrips
even
with your
hips

Keep your
weight off your
injured leg or
foot

Put crutches
about 1' in
front of you

you and swing your body forward
so you don't have to put weight
on the injured foot or leg. It helps
if you keep your eyes ahead in the
direction you are walking rather
than looking at your feet.

The easiest way to get up and
down stairs when you are on
crutches is to scoot on your bottom while holding the crutches in
one hand. If you want to try the
upright approach to go up stairs,
tuck the crutches under one arm
and use your hand on the
handrail to climb only with the
good foot. This assumes you have
the strength in the arm to hold
part of your weight while your
injured foot is raised behind you.
When going down you can hop,
one step at a time, on your good
foot while holding the crutches.

If there is no handrail, you can
try using the crutches to support
you while you climb up or down
stairs, but this can be tricky and
takes some strength. To go down,
move the crutches down first,
then your good leg, followed by
the injured one. To go up, first
move the good leg while the
crutches remain on the step.

A physical therapist can help you
learn the best techniques for
using crutches.

Walkers

Walkers provide more support
than either canes or crutches.
People with balance problems find

them useful as do people with hip replacements or arthritis where the goal is to keep as much weight off the lower extremities as possible. The type with four solid prongs and that you pick up is the most stable. The top of the walker should line up with the crease in your wrist when you stand up straight.

Using a walker requires taking small steps. Put the walker one step ahead of you on level ground and, with both hands, grip the top while you step off with your injured leg first, using your arms to keep as much of the weight off the injured side as possible. To sit, back up until your legs touch the chair.

Don't try climbing stairs or using an escalator with a walker.

People with good balance but who still need help when walking, such as people with cardiac conditions, may find a walker on wheels serves their needs. Cardiac patients may not have the strength to lift a walker as easily as push one. But a wheeled walker can slide out from under a person who has poor balance. Some walkers fold up so you can fit them in your car, but these tend to be more fragile.

To carry things with you while using the walker, try a fanny pack, a backpack, or an apron with pockets.

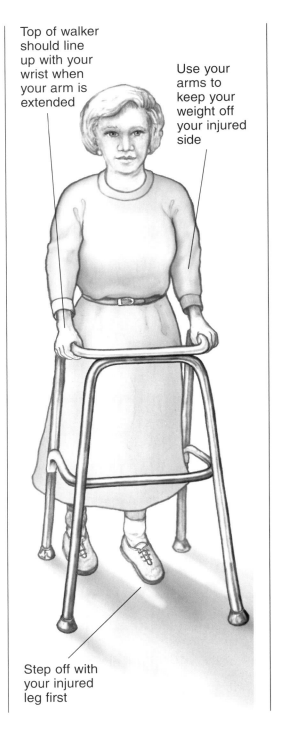

Top of walker should line up with your wrist when your arm is extended

Use your arms to keep your weight off your injured side

Step off with your injured leg first

ACHES AND PAINS OF PREGNANCY

Carrying the weight of a growing baby puts stress on a woman's body. It's not surprising, for example, that backaches and leg cramps are common complaints of pregnant women. Here are some suggestions for coping with these and other pregnancy-related pains.

Backache

The added weight centered at the front of a pregnant woman's body naturally puts extra strain on the back. The symptoms may be especially acute in women who gain more than the recommended amount of weight during pregnancy. A contributing factor is the pelvis. During pregnancy, its joints loosen in preparation for making enough room for the baby to eventually move down the birth canal. This slight change in the skeletal structure can throw your body a little off balance.

There are several things you can try to relieve the pain of a backache. Some women find that using a heating pad or a soaking in a warm bath provides temporary relief. But 3 to 4 hours later, the back may feel a bit stiff if the heat was sufficient to cause the muscles to swell. If that happens, try following the heat treatments with an application of a cold towel or ice pack.

Also, watch your posture and avoid standing with your stomach and pelvis thrust out. Wear low heeled or flat shoes. If you have to lift heavy loads, bend your knees and propel yourself up with your legs rather than bending at the waist. In fact, that should be the way you always lift things, not just when you're pregnant. Better still, avoid lifting heavy objects as much as possible, although if you already have a child, this may be difficult!

Avoid standing for long periods, although sitting for a long time can aggravate your back muscles, too. Instead of sinking into a soft sofa, pick a chair that provides firm support, especially in the back. A low footstool to elevate your feet can help make you more comfortable. Get up and move around every hour or so to stretch your muscles. If you are on a long car ride, stop for frequent breaks.

This might also be the time to invest in a firm mattress if your current one has seen better days. Or try putting a board between a too-soft mattress and the springs for better support. Find sleeping positions that take the load off your back. Many women are most comfortable lying on their left sides with a pillow under the leg

Relieving Back Strain

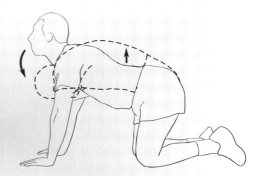

Try this exercise to relieve back strain. Get down on your hands and knees, keeping your back and head in a straight line like a tabletop. Then arch your spine like a cat, while tightening your buttocks and abdomen, and let your head drop toward the floor. Gradually return to your original position and repeat several times. Aerobic exercise such as walking can also help by increasing circulation and toning back and abdominal muscles, but consult your doctor before beginning an exercise program or continuing your pre-pregnancy workout. Some types of exercise are not appropriate during pregnancy, and women with high-risk pregnancies are even more restricted in what they can do.

that's on top. Some women will get temporary relief from massage therapy, chiropractic care, or even from acupuncture.

Exercises that strengthen the abdominal and lower back muscles and provide more support to your front ease the strain on your back. Finally, talk to your doctor if the pain becomes particularly troublesome. She may recommend you wear an undergarment for extra support or offer other suggestions. Do not take any medications unless your doctor approves. Remember that over-the-counter drugs, herbs, and supplements are considered "medications."

Also, consult your doctor if the pain migrates from your back into your thigh, leg, or foot or if you feel weakness or an altered sensation in your legs. These symptoms may be signs of sciatica, a distinctive type of pain that runs down from the lower back through the sciatic nerve. Some pregnant women experience sciatica because the pressure from the growing uterus can pinch this nerve. A heating pad and rest can help ease the symptoms.

Leg Cramps

Usually leg spasms occur when you are in bed at night. Frequent leg cramps can be a sign of a calcium shortage so your doctor may prescribe a supplement, especially if the problem becomes chronic and prevents you from getting enough sleep. Extra pressure from the growing fetus on nerves that extend into the legs may also be a cause. Standing on the leg can help. Or if you don't want to get up, try stretching your calf muscles by straightening your leg and bending your foot toward your face. After the cramp passes, massaging your leg can help it return to normal. If these pain remedies don't help, call your doctor, as this could be a sign of a circulation problem.

Hand Numbness and Tingling

Various parts of your body can swell during pregnancy. When this happens to the wrists, you may experience carpal tunnel syndrome. This condition is caused by swollen tendons in the wrist that put pressure on the median nerve running through a bony structure called the carpal tunnel. You may feel a painful tingling sensation or numbness in your hand and fingers. You've probably heard of it in connection with overuse injuries from manual work such as typing on a keyboard. In the case of pregnancy, it usually goes away after you give birth.

To relieve the sensations, try holding your hand above your head for a few minutes while opening and closing your fingers. Also, try to avoid sleeping on your

---

Relieving the Aches and Pains of Pregnancy

1. For backaches, watch your posture; avoid standing with your stomach and pelvis thrust out.

2. For leg cramps, try standing on the leg or if you are lying in bed stretch your calf muscles by straightening your leg and bending your foot toward your face.

3. For hand numbness or tingling, hold your hand above your head for a few minutes while opening and closing your fingers.

4. For rib pain while lying in bed, lift your hands and stretch upward to move your rib cage off the uterus.

---

hands. If the problem keeps you awake at night, consult your doctor who may recommend you wear a splint or try other remedies.

Rib Pain

Late in your pregnancy when your body has expanded up as well as out, you may feel rib pain when the baby is lying in a certain position. Try lifting your hands and stretching upward to move your rib cage off the uterus.

OSTEOPOROSIS

What It Is

You can't prevent bone loss as you age. It happens to everyone. But you can help prevent the most serious form of bone loss called osteoporosis, a potentially life-threatening condition that literally means "porous bone." Ten million Americans have it, and many more are at risk because they have low bone density.

Bone is a living tissue that is constantly remodeling—a process in which new bone tissue replaces old bone tissue that is absorbed by the body. It's because bones can generate new tissue that fractures are able to heal. But around age 35, your body starts to lose more bone mass than it replaces. This imbalance causes bone loss that continues throughout life. The loss accelerates in women after menopause due to a drop in estrogen, the female sex hormone that, among other things, helps maintain bone strength. After their bones have stopped growing, women may ultimately lose 30% to 50% of their bone mass over the course of their lives while men can lose 20% to 30%.

Eighty percent of the people who have osteoporosis are women. Caucasians or Asians have a higher incidence than people of other races. Although it usually strikes older people, it can affect people of any age. It's called a silent disease because you may not know you have it until you break a bone. The areas at highest risk for fractures associated with osteoporosis are the hip, spine, and wrist.

People with certain diseases such as rheumatoid arthritis, thyroid disease, diabetes, or liver ailments are at higher risk for osteoporosis than are those who take corticosteroids or anticonvulsant medications.

Signs and Symptoms

As bone thins and becomes fragile, small breaks can occur even from simple movements such as bending over or bumping into something. Because the spine and the hips are common spots for fractures in someone with osteoporosis, chronic pain can develop and become very debilitating. Complications of osteoporosis can be fatal in older people with broken hips (See p 38 for information on preventing falls.)

A common sign of osteoporosis is an elderly person who walks in a stooped position. This is due to small fractures in the spinal verte-

Risk Factors and Warning Signs

1. *A family history of osteoporosis*

2. *A thin or small frame*

3. *A low-calcium diet*

4. *A sedentary lifestyle*

5. *A history of smoking*

6. *Excessive use of alcohol*

brae that, instead of healing, collapse onto each other. The spine may curve, causing disfigurement, and you may get shorter.

Girls and women who don't have regular menstrual periods are at risk as they produce lower levels of estrogen. Eating disorders are a warning sign because they can contribute to irregular periods. Even frequent dieting can be a risk factor. While you lose and regain weight, you can lose bone density that you may not recoup later.

How to Detect It

Often, the first sign of osteoporosis in an older adult is a broken bone. At that point, the doctor will probably recommend a bone density test to assess bone strength and determine whether treatment is needed.

Various types of tests are used to screen for osteoporosis, using either a form of X-ray or ultrasound. The more expensive tests measure bone density in the hip or spine and are done in a specially equipped doctor's office or radiology facility. Simpler, inexpensive tests measure the bone in the heel or the finger. These are more widely available, sometimes even in pharmacies, and can help predict the likelihood of fracture. However, they aren't as accurate because they do not indicate the strength of hip or spinal bones, which may have less bone mass than the extremities.

Doctors differ on when bone density testing is needed, especially in individuals who haven't already experienced a fracture. Some suggest it for premenopausal women with risk factors or for all women when they reach menopause and for men over 65. Some doctors recommend testing to premenopausal women, whether they have risk factors or not, on the theory that if the bones are already showing signs of weakness, the patient will be more motivated to consume calcium and start exercising. Talk to your doctor about whether and when you should have a bone density test.

How to Treat It

 Doctors can't cure osteoporosis, but they can prescribe medications that can reduce bone loss and increase bone density. Some women take hormone replacement therapy (HRT), which treats menopausal symptoms such as hot flashes and also may help protect against osteoporosis. HRT in some menopausal women may increase the risk of breast cancer and cardiovascular disease. Other drugs are available to treat osteoporosis. Other women, who don't have those symptoms, opt for one of several drugs that have been approved to treat osteoporosis. If you've been diagnosed, discuss all options with your doctor.

When to Call the Doctor

Women who have reached menopause, or women or teens who aren't menstruating regularly, should consult their doctors about whether they should take HRT or other medications.

Prevention

There's a lot you can do to prevent osteoporosis. Two key steps are getting enough calcium and vitamin D in your diet (See p 19 for the "Healthy Bones Diet.") and ensuring that you incorporate weight-bearing exercises such as walking or jogging into your fitness routine. Maintaining a healthy lifestyle also includes avoiding risk factors such as smoking and excessive use of alcohol.

The earlier you start focusing on diet and exercise, the stronger your bones will be when you enter your later years and the less likely you will be to have brittle bones. That's why this message is especially important for children. You will reach most of your maximum bone mass by the time you are about 25 to 30. The more you have built up, the stronger your bones will be as you get older.

FIBROMYALGIA

What It Is

People with this chronic condition have widespread musculoskeletal pain and fatigue. The pain can be especially noticeable in "tender points" such as the neck, spine, shoul-

ders and hips (see figure). The American College of Rheumatology (ACR) estimates that three to six million Americans suffer from this condition, primarily women of childbearing age, although men and children sometimes are diagnosed with it.

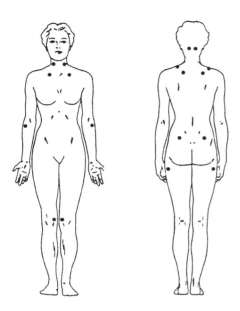

The cause is still unknown but research is underway to explore several promising theories. Some doctors think fibromyalgia may be triggered by a virus or other type of infection. Others speculate that it results from an injury that affects the central nervous system. Changes in muscle metabolism that decrease blood flow, causing muscles to become tired and weak, may also be a cause.

Because women are more likely to be diagnosed with fibromyalgia than men, hormones or other sex differences may provide clues. Recent government-funded studies indicate that fibromyalgia is associated with abnormally low levels of the hormone cortisol. Other scientists are researching whether there is a link between fibromyalgia and Lyme disease, an infection usually contracted from ticks.

Signs and Symptoms

Fibromyalgia is difficult to diagnose because the symptoms are similar to other disorders. The ACR has set criteria for doctors to use in diagnosis: If a patient has suffered widespread pain for more than 3 months, and if the pain is combined with tenderness in at least 11 of 18 specific tender point sites, the diagnosis may be fibromyalgia.

Some people with fibromyalgia also suffer from morning stiffness, sleep disturbances, irritable bowel syndrome, anxiety, and other symptoms.

When to Call the Doctor

If you have symptoms mirror those described above, call your doctor. You may be referred to an orthopaedic surgeon or to a rheumatologist.

How to Treat It

A combination approach of medication, exercise, physical therapy, and relaxation seems to work best. Aerobic exercise makes muscles stronger and less painful. Heat and massage are used for short-term pain relief. Medicines used include antidepressants to elevate mood, improve sleep and help patients relax. Teaching patients relaxation techniques also helps ease muscle tension. Acupuncture also has been used for pain relief.

Support groups for patients with fibromyalgia can be helpful for reassurance and to exchange information. Consult the Arthritis Foundation website for more information (www.arthritis.org).

LYME DISEASE

What It Is

Lyme disease is a bacterial infection that spreads to humans primarily through deer tick bites. About 16,000 infections are year are reported to the Centers for Disease Control and Prevention (CDC), and more than 90% of them come from 10 states: Maryland, Connecticut, Rhode Island, New York, Pennsylvania, New Jersey, Delaware, Massachusetts, Wisconsin, and Minnesota. It is also found on the West Coast, especially in northern California.

Lyme disease is easily treated with antibiotics if caught in the early stages but can lead to arthritis or other problems later if not diagnosed promptly.

Diagnosis is tricky because some of the symptoms of Lyme disease mimic other illnesses.

Signs and Symptoms

Approximately 80% of infected people have a rash that looks like a red bull's eye at the site of the bite, usually within 7 to 14 days. The rash gradually expands and can grow to cover a large area of the thigh, groin, trunk or armpits. The rash usually isn't painful but may feel warm. You may also have flu-like symptoms including fever, chills, headache, fatigue, swollen lymph nodes, and muscle and joint pain.

Just because you have a rash at the site of a tick bite, however, doesn't mean you have Lyme disease. Often people have allergic

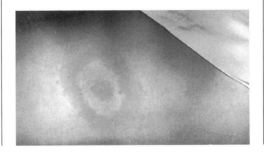

reactions to tick saliva. The difference is that an allergic rash usually appears within hours of the bite, doesn't get bigger, and disappears in a few days.

Some people with Lyme disease never get a rash. The first and only sign may show up months or even years later as arthritis involving brief bouts of pain and swelling in one or more large joints, especially the knee. The disease can also cause nervous system abnormalities including numbness and pain in various muscles.

When to Call the Doctor

Call if you have the rash or some of the other symptoms described above and have experienced a tick bite in the recent past. Any symptoms of arthritis should be checked by your doctor.

How to Treat It

Early treatment with antibiotics usually provides a full and rapid recovery. Antibiotics are also effective at treating later stage Lyme disease but must be taken longer.

Prevention

Fortunately, only a tiny fraction of bites result in Lyme disease, and there's a lot you can do to prevent tick

Why Lyme Disease?

Lyme disease gets its name from Lyme, Connecticut, where the illness was first identified in 1975 after a mysterious outbreak of arthritis among children living in the area.

bites. Before walking in wooded areas or tall grass, spray your clothes and exposed skin (except your face) with bug repellent containing DEET. For added protection, wear long-sleeved shirts tucked into slacks. Tuck the ends of the slacks into your socks.

When you come back inside, throw the clothes in the washer and dryer and inspect your body. If you find a tick, the CDC recommends that you remove it with tweezers; grasping it as close to the skin as possible and pulling straight back. The CDC says prompt removal is important because it usually takes 2 days for the tick to transmit the infection after attaching to the skin.

A vaccine is available but is only recommended for people at high risk, such as those whose jobs expose them to wooded areas. More research is needed to determine the long-term benefits of the vaccine.

GOUT

What It Is

Gout is a very painful metabolic condition caused by crystal deposits that lodge in joints and cause inflammation. The crystals form as the result of an excess of uric acid in the body. The joint at the base of the big toe is often the site, but joints in the foot, ankle, knee, and elbow can sometimes be involved, too.

Usually, uric acid that forms in the body is excreted in urine. If there is too much for the kidneys to excrete, the acid accumulates in the blood and forms crystals that find their way into the joints. The tendency for gout to develop is sometimes hereditary, but it can also be the result of a uric acid imbalance caused by drinking too much alcohol or eating too much protein-rich food. Kidney diseases or certain medications can also result in too much uric acid. Being overweight is an additional risk factor.

The first episode usually affects one joint and lasts only a few days. That may be the only case of gout you'll ever have. But often, a second episode occurs, although perhaps not for months or years. After this, you'll usually have more episodes with increasing frequency and more joints affected unless you seek treatment to prevent recurrences.

Signs and Symptoms

An episode of gout begins with severe pain in a joint that comes without warning, often at night. The pain becomes excruciating; if it's your toe that's affected, you might not even want the weight of a bed sheet on it. The skin over the joint will appear red or purplish and shiny and will be hot to the touch. You may also have a low-grade fever and chills and generally feel sick. If you are under 30, the symptoms tend to be even more severe than if you are older.

If left untreated, episodes of gout become more frequent, last longer, and can cause permanent joint deformity.

Gout Strikes Men First

Men can have an attack of gout at any time after puberty, but women don't usually have it until after menopause. In men, gout is more common than in women, with the first episode usually occurring in middle age.

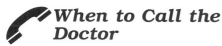

When to Call the Doctor

Call the doctor if you think you have gout.

How to Treat It

Even though the problem should go away on its own in a few days, the doctor can prescribe an anti-inflammatory pain medication that will ease the symptoms faster and can advise you regarding dietary restrictions to prevent recurrences. The affected joint may need to be aspirated (drained) so that the doctor can analyze some of the fluid for uric acid crystals to confirm the diagnosis.

You may not need further treatment unless you have repeat episodes. At that point your doctor may prescribe medication that can prevent additional episodes or at least reduce their frequency.

Prevention

To prevent recurrences, drink lots of water or other nonalcoholic liquids to flush the uric acid out of your system. Cut down on your consumption of alcoholic beverages and protein-rich foods. People who are overweight and have gout find that losing weight helps reduce their uric acid levels.

RHEUMATOID ARTHRITIS

While it's true that arthritis is the leading cause of disability in the United States, it's a myth that arthritis is an inevitable part of aging that must be endured. Doctors and patients have many options for treatment available to reduce the pain and disability of arthritis. Although there are more than 100 different types of arthritis, the two most common kinds are rheumatoid arthritis (RA) and osteoarthritis (OA). Currently, there is no cure for these,

although research is ongoing to find cures as well as more effective treatments.

What It Is

RA is a disease in which the lining of the joints (synovium) produces chemicals that attack and destroy the joint surfaces.

The hands and feet are commonly affected, but larger joints such as the hips, knees, and elbows also

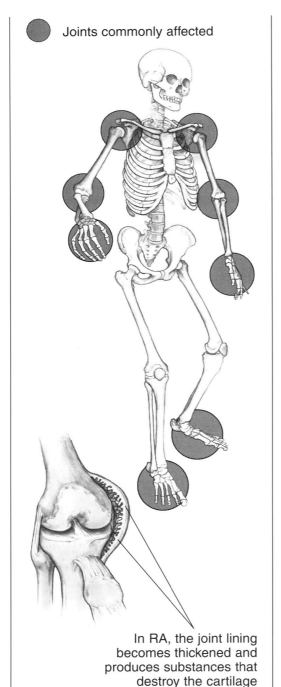

Joints commonly affected

In RA, the joint lining becomes thickened and produces substances that destroy the cartilage lining of the joint.

can be affected. Multiple joints may be involved, and usually there is symmetry, meaning for example, that both hands or both feet are involved rather than just one. This symmetry is distinct from other types of arthritis such as OA and is one of the ways RA is diagnosed.

RA affects people of every age, although we often hear more about juvenile RA. Typically, RA is first diagnosed in middle age, with more than 70% of patients over 30 years old. RA affects two to three times more women than men.

Although RA isn't inherited, scientists think some people have certain genes that make them more susceptible, and that the genes are activated by a trigger such as a viral infection or other environmental factor. The fact that women are more affected than men suggests hormones also play a role.

Signs and Symptoms

The inflammation that is characteristic of RA causes swelling, pain, and stiffness, even when the joint isn't moving. RA can lead to an inability to stretch or bend the joint (called a contracture) and joint deformity. You may feel warmth in the joint, and some people develop nodules or lumps at affected sites in the body. You may also have general symptoms such as fever, loss of appetite, little energy, and anemia (low red blood cell count).

To diagnose RA, your doctor will use blood tests and X-rays, as well as a physical exam and your medical history.

How to Treat It

Some medications are used to treat the symptoms. Others help slow the progression of the disease. Your doctor may recommend you take both types. Nonsteroidal anti-inflammatory drugs (NSAIDs) such as aspirin and ibuprofen help relieve pain and inflammation. Glucosamine and chondroitin sulfate are over-the-counter supplements that are considered potentially helpful and are relatively safer than NSAIDs. Many herbals are also thought to have mild anti-inflammatory benefits, but none have been shown to have a significant benefit. Disease-modifying, anti-rheumatic drugs (DMARDs) include methotrexate, sulfasalazine, and gold salt injections. Corticosteroids, taken orally, topically, or by injection, are also used to treat symptoms in some cases. Corticosteroids are strong drugs with some side effects such as harming articular cartilage. For this reason, doctors limit the frequency and number of injections administered in an arthritic joint.

Although RA causes pain and fatigue, you should try to balance rest with a program of appropriate exercise since movement helps reduce pain and improves flexibility, strength, and endurance. In particular, doctors recommend exercises such as swimming that don't put extra stress on the joints. Physical therapists can teach patients the right ways to exercise and may use other techniques such as heat therapy to decrease stiffness. Patients can be taught new methods of performing daily activities that put less stress on joints. For example, there are special tools that help arthritis patients open jars without straining their hands or pick things up from the floor so they can avoid bending over. Relaxation therapy, in which patients learn to release muscle tension, can also help ease pain. A well-balanced diet also helps keep patients with arthritis healthy and helps them manage their weight. Gaining too many pounds puts additional stress on already sore joints.

Using a cane, crutches, or a walker can take some of the weight off an arthritic knee or hip. Shoe inserts (called orthotics) can ease the pain of an arthritic foot. Splints or braces, such as on the hand or wrist, are sometimes used to give weakened joints time to rest.

When other methods fail, doctors sometimes recommend surgery to relieve arthritis symptoms. This can include removing the damaged joint lining, realigning the joint, total joint replacement, or fusion of the bones so the joint no longer moves and causes pain.

Kids Have Arthritis, Too

The childhood version of this disease is called juvenile rheumatoid arthritis (JRA). In most cases, the symptoms are mild and don't cause progressive joint disease, although in serious cases there can be joint and tissue damage and problems with bone growth and development. Most kids eventually grow out of it.

As with adult RA, scientists believe some children have genes that put them at risk and that the disease is triggered by a virus or exposure to something else in the environment.

Signs include joints that are painful in the morning but feel better in the afternoon. You might notice a morning limp if a knee is affected, and the joint may feel warm to the touch. The child may not complain of pain but may appear unwell and may even have a high fever or light pink rash briefly. Sometimes lymph nodes in the neck or other places become swollen.

Some children with JRA also have a related eye problem called iridocyclitis, which is treatable by an eye specialist (ophthalmologist). The main symptom is pain during exposure to bright light, although some children with the eye problem don't have this symptom. If it is not treated, iridocyclitis can lead to irreversible eye damage.

The symptoms of JRA are usually treated with medication and physical therapy to help the child maintain a normal life until the symptoms subside. Sometimes splints are used, especially on the hands to prevent finger and wrist contracture. In a few cases, surgery is needed to repair damaged joints.

OSTEOARTHRITIS

While it's true that arthritis is the leading cause of disability in the United States, it's a myth that arthritis is an inevitable part of aging that must be endured. Doctors and patients have many options for treatment available to reduce the pain and disability of arthritis. Although there are more than 100 different types of arthritis, the two most common kinds are rheumatoid arthritis (RA) and osteoarthritis (OA). Currently, there is no cure for these, although research is ongoing to find cures as well as more effective treatments.

What It Is

? OA is sometimes called "wear-and-tear" arthritis because the condition involves the wearing away of cartilage, the cushioning material attached to the ends of bones, which cuts down on friction. As we age, the constant movement of joints makes the cartilage thinner. Unlike RA, which is a disease that affects multiple joints and joint pairs, OA can affect a single joint, often a large weight-bearing one such as the hip or knee.

Younger people can have OA in a joint, too, as a result of overuse. A baseball pitcher can have it in the elbow and a floor tile layer

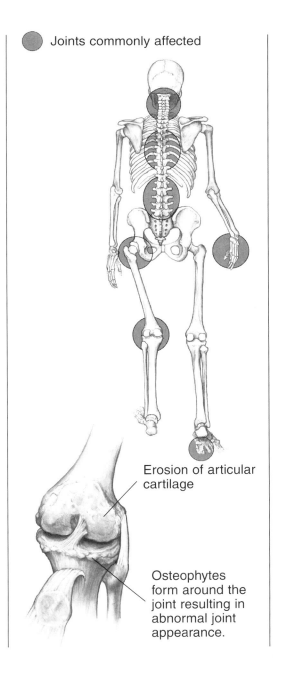

Joints commonly affected

Erosion of articular cartilage

Osteophytes form around the joint resulting in abnormal joint appearance.

may have it in a knee. Sometimes OA develops in a joint as the result of a fracture that didn't healed properly.

Signs and Symptoms

Many people never experience symptoms from OA but for others, joints can become inflamed, swollen, and painful. Sometimes bony growths called spurs develop in the joints, too.

Complementary and Alternative Medicine

Patients suffering from the pain of arthritis sometimes turn to what's called complementary or alternative medicine (sometimes abbreviated as CAM). Examples include meditation, relaxation therapy, massage, acupuncture, and dietary or herbal supplements, sometimes called nutriceuticals. In this latter category, two over-the-counter supplements, glucosamine and chondroitin sulfate, have received much attention. Both are natural substances found in the body; the types sold in health food stores are derived from animal products.

The federal government is engaged in a long-term study of the effectiveness of these compounds, but preliminary studies by other scientists have shown these supplements may help relieve the pain of OA. There is some evidence that they slow the degenerative process or repair damage, however. Further study is needed to determine their effectiveness at pain relief, at what doses and for how long a period of time.

One problem with taking glucosamine and chondroitin sulfate is that the US Food and Drug Administration (FDA) is not responsible for confirming the purity, potency, or quality of various brands of nutritional supplements, so you can't be sure the bottle you buy actually contains what the labels claim. That's why, if you decide to try these supplements, you should stick with name brands from reputable manufacturers. Look for USP on the label; this indicates that the product conforms to quality standards of the US Pharmacopeia, a voluntary compliance organization.

If you decide to try nutritional supplements, don't stop your current regimen of diet, exercise, medication, or other therapies. Also, because these supplements aren't appropriate for all forms of arthritis and because they aren't recommended for some people—such as those with diabetes—talk to your doctor before taking them. Many physicians are open to complementary treatments and can help you make decisions about what to try.

How to Treat It

Some of the same treatments used for RA are also used to treat OA: rest balanced with appropriate exercises to keep muscles above the joint strong, use of braces, and applications of heat and ice. Heat makes the joint feel better temporarily but may make the joint feel stiffer several hours later. Ice is not as soothing as heat but does decrease inflammation and thereby eases pain. Try applying heat for 10 to 15 minutes, followed by ice. Some people try this trick for fast relief: soak a face cloth in water and put it in the freezer. Later you can wrap the affected area with the frozen cloth.

Other treatments include medications and various types of surgical repair. Total joint replacements can be very effective, and new surgical methods are being developed to use cartilage grafts to replace isolated areas of wear within a joint.

PHYSICAL THERAPY AND REHABILITATION BASICS

Treatment of musculoskeletal injuries or diseases usually includes specialized exercises and sometimes other types of physical therapy to improve the functioning of the body part. If you only need some simple rehabilitation exercises, your doctor or nurse may teach them to you or may provide a handout with instructions to use at home. If a more complex rehabilitation program of exercise is needed, the doctor may refer you to a physical therapist. This would be true for example, if you need to be watched to make sure you are performing the exercises correctly. If you've had surgery, you'll probably need a physical therapist to regularly monitor the progress of your rehabilitation and then adjust your exercise program accordingly.

Here's a brief guide to exercise and other treatment methods. Examples of simple stretching and strengthening exercises, along with tips for weight training, are provided on pp 65-84. They also can be downloaded from www.aaos.org/almanac.

Strengthening Exercises

After an injury that has caused a part of the body to become temporarily immobilized, muscles can become weak. Strength training, also called weight training, builds up the muscles and can help prevent further injury. For example, an injury to the knee joint is less likely to recur if the thigh and calf muscles are strong. Strength training involves adding resistance to the body's natural movements in order to make the movements more difficult and encourage the muscles to become stronger.

Initially, the weight of your limb may be all the resistance you need. Gradually, you can incorporate more resistance using various types of equipment such as weights or a resistance machine as part of your rehabilitation.

During physical therapy, you may hear the terms isometrics and isokinetics. There are two types of strength training exercises.

Isometric exercises are static in that the muscles don't change length during them. Isometrics are often the first type of exercise recommended following a serious injury. You tense the muscle for some seconds and then let it relax. You might do this by lifting the limb while it is straight or push against an immovable object, for example.

Isokinetic exercises are referred to as dynamic because in these movements, the muscle lengthens or shortens as the body part bends and straightens.

Stretching Exercises

Lack of movement following an injury can make muscles tighten up. Stretching exercises make the muscles more flexible and also help prevent injuries in the future. By increasing the blood flow to the muscles, they become warm and looser. This is why performing stretching exercises before engaging in strenuous physical activity is called warming up. Stretching exercises are often combined with a program of strengthening exercises.

Staying relaxed and breathing slowly are important for proper stretching. You should not feel pain.

Range-of-Motion Exercises

Injuries or disease sometimes makes joints less flexible than they once were, which in turn prevents a body part, an arm or knee for example, from moving as far as it normally would. The way to increase mobility is through range-of-motion exercises designed to stretch that part of the body. Your doctor or physical therapist can recommend specific range of motion exercises appropriate for your particular condition.

Cryotherapy

This is a fancy name for applying ice. The cold temperature slows circulation to reduce internal bleeding. This in turn reduces swelling, inflammation, and pain. It is usually one of the first treatments recommended for a musculoskeletal injury. You don't actually apply ice directly to the skin as this can cause frostbite. Instead, use a commercially available ice pack, ice cubes wrapped in a thin towel or a bag of frozen vegetables. The usual recommendation is to apply ice for about 20 minutes every 2 to 3 hours for the first 2 or 3 days following an injury.

Thermotherapy

This is a fancy name for applying heat. After the first 2 or 3 days, when icing has stopped the bleeding, swelling, and inflammation, you may find it helpful to apply heat. Heat helps relieve stiffness and stimulates the circulation of blood which speeds healing.

You can use a standard heating pad, but dry heat isn't as effective as moist heat—from showers, hot baths, or whirlpools—that penetrates deeper into the tissue. Moist heating pads are also available for use at home.

Caution: Heating pads can burn your skin if you don't exercise care in using them. Follow the instructions that come with the pad and never sleep while using one.

Contrast Baths

Some people find relief from symptoms by using contrast baths. The injured extremity is submerged first in ice water for about 30 seconds and then plunged into water that is as warm as you can tolerate (usually about 104°F) for 30 seconds. Continue alternating cold and hot for about 5 minutes and end in the cold water.

Ultrasound

With this treatment, high-frequency sound waves applied to the injured area cause the tissues to vibrate. This generates heat, increases circulation, and speeds healing. It can also relieve pain, reduce muscle spasms, and increase range of motion.

Treatments are usually administered by a physical therapist or an athletic trainer. The instrument looks like a hand-held vibrator that is rubbed over the affected body part. An application of a gel makes the instrument glide easily over the skin. A typical treatment session lasts 10 to 15 minutes, repeated two to three times per week until the symptoms are relieved. Ultrasound is used for a variety of conditions, especially tendinitis, bursitis, and joint and muscle strains. It is very safe when given by a qualified medical professional.

Transcutaneous Electric Nerve Stimulation (TENS)

Electrical stimulation applied to a soft-tissue injury is used to ease chronic pain. The idea is that the central nervous system can only let in so much input. If you flood it with impulses, the nervous system can't perceive the pain impulses as readily. You typically wear a portable, battery-operated device called a TENS unit which sends low-voltage electrical impulses to the injured area. The impulses are sent via the nerve endings to the brain, blocking the pain signals. The unit can be worn while you are at home, either intermittently or throughout the day. You control the intensity of the stimulation, and you will hardly feel the impulses. Many patients find that a TENS unit reduces their need for pain medication. You can rent a TENS unit either through your doctor's office, hospital or physical therapist. Patients who need them for a long time, such a those with chronic back pain, sometimes opt to purchase the unit.

Complementary and Alternative Medicine Devices

Complementary and alternative medicine (CAM) includes techniques and devices that are not widely accepted by conventional medicine. Some techniques are promising, and with good scientific research, may become more widely accepted. Others, however, offer little benefit beyond their "mind over matter" or placebo effects. Copper bracelets, for example, have no demonstrated benefit for the wearer.

Today magnets are widely promoted as devices that will relieve the symptoms of arthritis and other musculoskeletal conditions. Much research has been devoted to identifying whether magnets have any effect on musculoskeletal symptoms. To date, there is no widely accepted research that documents any benefit of magnets.

Thus, a good rule of thumb is to exercise healthy skepticism of any claim that seems too good to be true. If you are considering using some device or modality, ask your doctor first. Doctors are educated scientists who are trained to evaluate evidence related to treatment alternatives.

Sports Warm-Up/General Stretching Exercises

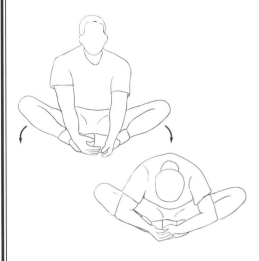

Seat Straddle Lotus

Sit down on the floor, place the soles of your feet together, and drop your knees toward the floor. Place your forearms on the inside of your knees and gently push your knees to the floor. Lean forward, bringing your chin to your feet. Hold for 5 seconds. Repeat 3 to 6 times.

Seat Side Straddle

Sit down on the floor with your legs spread apart. Place both of your hands on the same ankle and bring your chin to your knee. Hold for 5 seconds. Alternate from side to side. Repeat 3 to 6 times.

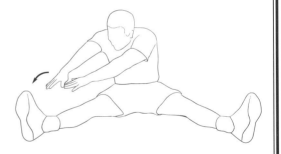

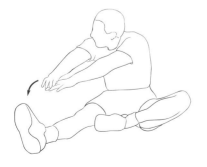

Modified Seat Side Straddle

To modify this exercise, bend one leg as shown.

Sports Warm-Up/General Stretching Exercises

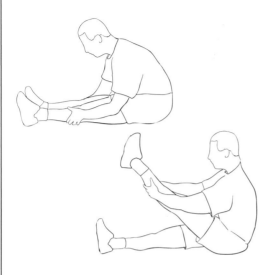

Leg Stretch

Sit down on the floor with your legs straight and your hands on the backs of your calves. Slowly lift and pull each leg individually toward your ear, keeping your back straight. Hold for 5 seconds. Alternate from side to side. Repeat each leg 3 to 6 times. You can slightly bend the leg not being stretched if it's more comfortable.

Sitting Rotation Stretch

Sit down on the floor with both legs straight. Cross one leg over the other and rotate your body toward the crossed leg and back in the other direction. Hold for 30 seconds. Repeat in the opposite direction, switching crossed legs. Repeat 3 times in each direction.

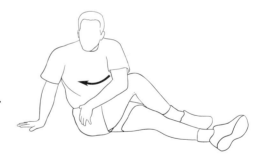

Knee to Chest

Lie on your back on the floor with your knees bent and heels flat on the floor. Grasp one knee and bring it up to your chest as far as it will go, then lower your leg back to the floor. Do the same thing with your other leg. Next use both legs together. Continue to alternate until you do 10 of each. Work up to 3 sets of 10.

Sports Warm-Up/General Stretching Exercises

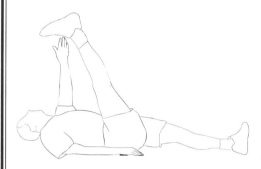

Leg Cross-over

Lie down on the floor with your legs spread and your arms out to your sides. Bring your right toe to your left hand, keeping your leg straight. Hold for 5 seconds. Alternate from side to side. Repeat each leg 3 to 6 times. You may slightly bend the leg on the floor if it's more comfortable.

Cross-over Stand

Stand with your legs crossed. Keep your feet close together and your legs straight. Slowly bend forward toward your toes. Hold for 5 seconds. Repeat with the opposite leg crossed in front.

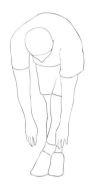

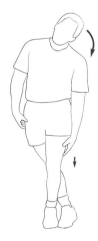

Iliotibial Band Stretch

Stand with your weight evenly distributed, next to a wall for support if desired. Cross one leg behind the other. Lean your hip toward the wall until you feel a stretch on the outside of the leg. Hold for 10 seconds and then relax. Perform 3 sets of 10 on each side, 3 times a day.

Sports Warm-Up/General Stretching Exercises

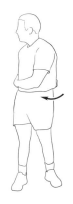

Torso Rotation

Stand with your weight evenly distributed and your feet shoulder-width apart, or sit with proper back posture. Rotate your torso to the right as far as possible. Hold for 3 seconds. Alternate from side to side. Repeat 10 times on each side.

Side Stretch

Stand with your weight evenly distributed and your feet shoulder-width apart. Place one hand at your side and the other above your head, leaning to the opposite side. Hold for 15 seconds, repeating three times on each side.

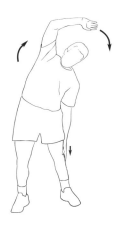

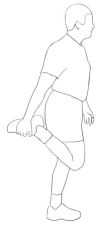

Standing Quadriceps Stretch

Stand supported. Bend your knee up toward your buttock and grasp your ankle. Pull up gently and hold for 5 seconds. Repeat with the opposite leg.

Sports Warm-Up/General Stretching Exercises

Prone Quadriceps Stretch

Lie down on the floor with your arms at your sides and your legs straight out. Bend your knee up toward your buttock and grasp your ankle. Pull up gently and hold for 5 seconds. Repeat with the opposite leg.

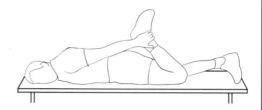

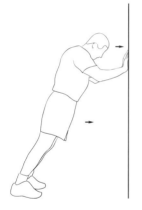

Heel Cord Stretch

Stand 3 feet from the wall with your feet pointed straight ahead. Lower your hips to the wall without raising your heels off the floor. Hold for 5 seconds. Repeat 3 to 6 times.

2-Person Hamstring Stretch

Lie down on the floor with your legs straight. Your partner then brings one leg up only to the point of tightness and resists while you try to push your leg down. Relax while your partner pushes you leg farther until it feels tight again. Repeat with the opposite leg. You may also slightly bend the leg on the floor if it's more comfortable.

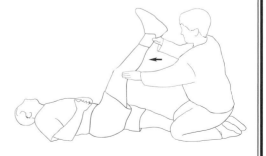

Sports Warm-Up/General Stretching Exercises

2-Person Prone Quadriceps Stretch

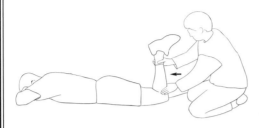

Lie down on your stomach with your legs straight. Your partner then grasps your lower leg and bends it until you feel a stretch on the front of the thigh. As your partner is holding your leg, push against your partner for 5 seconds. Relax while your partner bends your leg again until you feel another stretch. Repeat with the opposite leg.

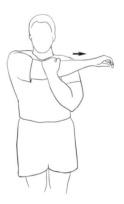

Cross-over Arm Stretch

Grasp the elbow of the injured arm with your opposite hand and pull the arm across the front of your chest. Hold for 5 seconds and then relax. Perform 25 times 3 times a day.

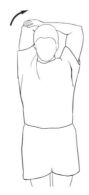

Overhead Arm Stretch

Raise your injured arm above your head, as high toward the ear as possible, and bend the elbow with the palm up. Use your opposite hand to help pull the arm toward the ear. Hold for 5 seconds and then relax. Perform 25 times 3 times a day.

Shoulder & Elbow Strengthening Exercises

Abduction

Stand with your weight evenly distributed, with a light weight (up to 5 lb) in
the hand of your injured shoulder.
Raise your arm out to the side of your
body only to the level of your shoulder, with your thumb pointed straight
ahead. Work up to 5 sets of 10, two to
three times a day.

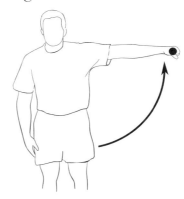

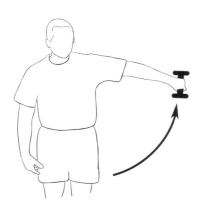

Internal Rotation

Stand with your weight evenly distributed, with a light weight (up to 5 lb) in
the hand of your injured shoulder.
Hold the weight with a pronated grip.
Raise your arm out to the side of your
body only to the level of your shoulder, with your thumb pointed down.
Work up to 5 sets of 10, two to three
times a day.

Prone Horizontal Abduction

Stand bent at the waist with your
uninjured side supported by leaning
on a table with your injured extremity hanging should straight to the
floor. With a light weight (up to 5 lb),
raise your arm out to the side with
your thumb up and hand at eye
level. Work up to 5 sets of 10, two
to three times a day.

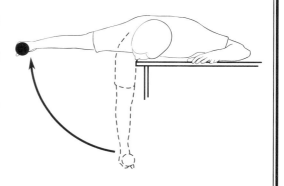

Shoulder & Elbow Strengthening Exercises

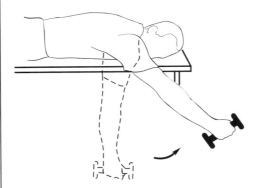

Prone External Rotation

Stand bent at the waist with your uninjured side supported by leaning on a table with your injured extremity hanging should straight to the floor. With a light weight (up to 5 lb), raise your arm forward to level with the table. Work up to 5 sets of 10, two to three times a day.

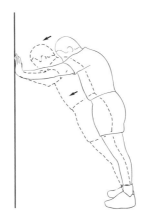

Wall Push-up

Stand next to a wall and perform a push-up in the standard way. On reaching the top position of the movement, roll your shoulder blades forward and hold for 5 seconds. Work toward performing standard push-ups on the floor.

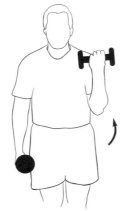

Elbow Flexion

Sit or stand with your weight evenly distributed with your injured arm at your side. Holding a light weight in the hand of your injured arm, bend your elbow toward your shoulder, hold for 5 seconds and then relax. Work up to 5 sets of 10, two to three times a day.

Shoulder & Elbow Strengthening Exercises

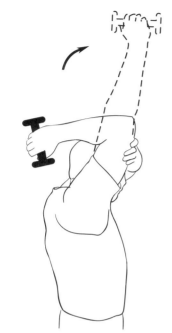

Elbow Extension

Sit or stand with your weight evenly distributed with your injured arm raised overhead and your opposite arm supporting your elbow. Holding a light weight in the hand of your injured arm, straighten your elbow overhead, hold for 5 seconds then bend your elbow and relax. Work up to 5 sets of 10, two to three times a day.

Caution: You must have some triceps strength to control the weight. If you do not have adequate triceps strength, begin with the weight lower than shoulder height.

Wrist & Elbow Strengthening Exercises

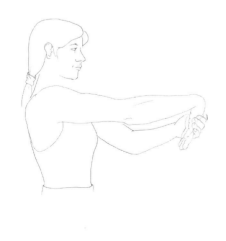

Wrist Extension

Extend your arm and hand out and flex your wrist so your fingers point down. Use your opposite hand to apply gentle pressure to the back of the hand to push it back as far as it will go. Hold for 10 to 15 seconds. Repeat three times.

Wrist & Elbow Strengthening Exercises

Wrist Flexion

Extend your arm and hand out as if you are signaling someone to "stop" (Fingers can point up or down). Place your opposite hand across the palm and gently push your hand back as far as it will go. Hold for 10 to 15 seconds. Repeat three times.

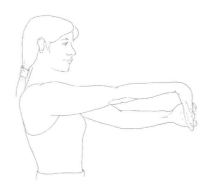

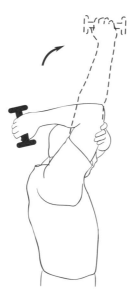

Elbow Extension

Sit or stand with your weight evenly distributed with your injured arm raised overhead and your opposite arm supporting your elbow. Holding a light weight in the hand of your injured arm, straighten your elbow overhead, hold for 5 seconds then bend your elbow and relax. Work up to 5 sets of 10, two to three times a day.

Caution: You must have some triceps strength to control the weight. If you do not have adequate triceps strength, begin with the weight lower than shoulder height.

Wrist Extension

Sit with your forearm supported on a table, with your hand off the edge, palm facing down to the floor. Holding a light weight in the hand of your injured arm, bend your wrist so that you lower your hand as far as possible and then curl it up as high as possible. Hold for 5 seconds, and then relax your wrist. Work up to 5 sets of 10, two to three times a day.

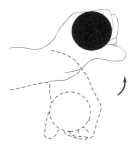

Wrist & Elbow Strengthening Exercises

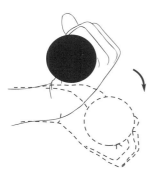

Wrist Flexion

Sit with your forearm supported on a table, with your hand off the edge, palm facing up. Holding a light weight in the hand of your injured arm, bend your wrist so that you lower your hand as far as possible and then curl it up as high as possible. Hold for 5 seconds, and then relax your wrist. Work up to 5 sets of 10, two to three times a day.

Wrist Supination

Sit with your forearm supported on a table, with your hand off the edge, wrist in a neutral position. Holding a light weight in the hand of your injured arm, roll your wrist into full supination. Hold for 5 seconds, and then relax your wrist. Work up to 5 sets of 10, two to three times a day.

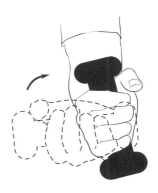

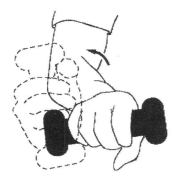

Wrist Pronation

Sit with your forearm supported on a table, with your hand off the edge, wrist in a neutral position. Holding a light weight in the hand of your injured arm, roll your wrist into pronation as far as possible. Hold for 5 seconds, and then relax your wrist. Work up to 5 sets of 10, two to three times a day.

Knee Range-of-Motion Exercises—Early Rehabilitation

Heel Slide

Lie on the floor with your legs straight out. Slide your heel up toward your buttocks, flexing your knee as much as possible. Hold it for 5 seconds, then slowly straighten your leg. Perform 3 sets of 10, three times a day.

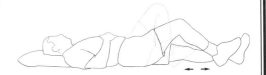

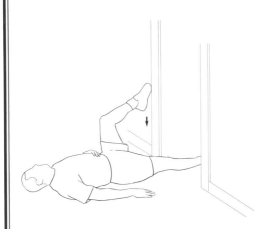

Wall Slide

Lie on your back in a doorway, with one leg supported by the wall. Put your foot up on the wall and then let it gently slide down the wall. Hold it for 5 seconds, then slowly straighten your leg. Perform 3 sets of 10, three times a day.

Knee Flexion

Lie face down on the floor or on a bed with your legs together. Slowly flex your knee up toward your buttocks and then lower it. You may also use rubber tubing to do this exercise. Ask your doctor how many repetitions per day.

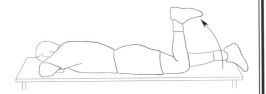

Knee Range-of-Motion Exercises—Early Rehabilitation

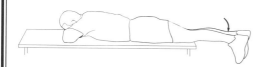

Knee Extension—Passive Stretching

Lie face down on the floor or on a bed with your thighs supported just above the knee. Gravity pulls your knee down (into extension) as you relax. Ask your doctor how many repetitions per day. Also, your doctor may advise you to add light weights to your ankles to increase the stretch.

Knee Extension

Sit in a chair with your injured leg propped as shown. Gravity pulls your knee down (into extension) as you relax. Ask your doctor how many repetitions per day.

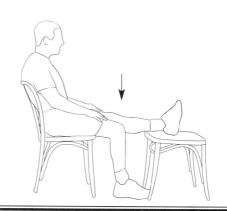

Knee Strengthening Exercises—Early Rehabilitation

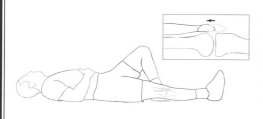

Quadriceps Strengthening

Lie on the floor with the injured leg straight out and the other bent. Squeeze your thigh muscle for 10 seconds and then release it. Ask your doctor how many repetitions per day.

Knee Strengthening Exercises—Early Rehabilitation

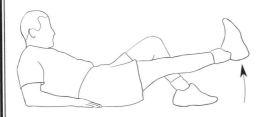

Straight Leg Raise

Lie down on the floor with your injured leg straight and the other leg bent. Tighten the thigh muscle of the straight leg and slowly raise it 6" to 10" off of the floor. Hold it for 5 seconds. Work up to 3 sets of 10.

Abduction

Lie down on the floor on the side of your uninjured leg with both legs straight. Raise the injured leg 6" to 8" off of the floor. Hold it for 5 seconds. Lower the leg and rest for 2 seconds. Work up to 3 sets of 10.

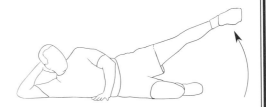

Adduction

Lie down on the floor on the side of your injured leg with both legs straight. Cross the uninjured leg in front of the injured one. Raise the injured leg 6" to 8" off of the floor. Hold it for 5 seconds. Lower the leg and rest for 2 seconds. Work up to 3 sets of 10.

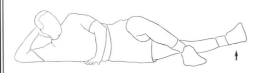

Straight Leg Raise (Prone)

Lie down on the floor on your stomach with your legs straight. Extend the knee, then tighten the hamstrings of the injured leg. Raise that leg behind you as far as you can. Hold it for 5 seconds. Lower the leg and rest 2 seconds. Work up to 3 sets of 10.

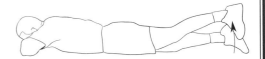

Knee Strengthening Exercises—Early Rehabilitation

Hamstring Curls

Stand on a flat surface, with your weight evenly distributed. Hold the back of a chair or onto a wall for balance. Raise the heel of your uninjured leg toward the ceiling. Hold it for 5 seconds and then relax. Perform 5 sets of 10, three times a day.

Note: This exercise also can be done seated, so you do not have to balance yourself while standing.

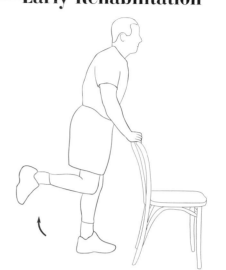

Knee Strengthening Exercises—Advanced Rehabilitation

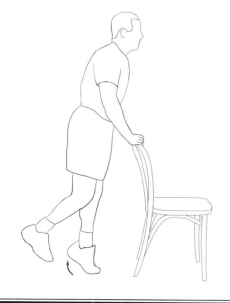

Calf Raises

Stand on a flat surface, with your weight evenly distributed. Hold the back of a chair or onto a wall for balance. Raise the heel of your uninjured leg off of the floor as high as you can, using your body weight as resistance. Work up to 3 sets of 10.

Knee Strengthening Exercises— Advanced Rehabilitation

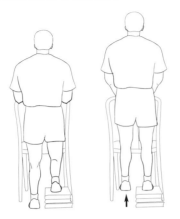

Side Step Up

Stand sideways with the involved leg toward the step. Place the foot of that leg upon the step and lift yourself up while pushing off with the toe of the uninjured leg. Progress to standing on the heel of the uninjured leg and lifting yourself up with no push-off. Perform 5 sets of 10, three times a day

Wall Slide

Stand with your back against a wall and your feet about 1 foot from the wall. Tuck your pelvis under so your low back is flat against the wall. Stop when your knees are bent 90°. Hold for 5 seconds and then relax. Work up to 3 sets of 10.

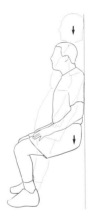

Forward Lunge

Bend your left knee and put your right leg forward at a right angle. Lunge forward, keeping your back straight. You should feel a slight stretch on the left groin area. Hold for 5 seconds. Repeat with the opposite leg.

Knee Strengthening Exercises—Advanced Rehabilitation

Side Lunge

Stand with your legs apart. Bend your left knee and lean toward the left, keeping your back straight and your right leg straight. Hold for 5 seconds. Repeat with the opposite leg.

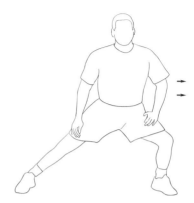

Back Strengthening Exercises

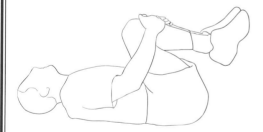

Knees to Chest

Lie down on the floor with your knees bent. Grasp the tops of your knees and bring them slowly to your chest, rocking gently. Repeat 3 to 6 times.

Pelvic Tilt

Lie on your back on the floor with your knees bent and feet flat on the floor. Tighten your stomach muscles and tilt your pelvis so your lower back becomes flat against the floor. Hold this position for 5 seconds and then relax. Repeat 10 times.

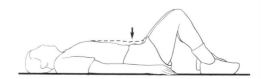

Back Strengthening Exercises

Knee to Chest

Lie on your back on the floor with your knees bent and feet flat on the floor. Grasp one knee and bring it up to your chest as far as it will go, then lower your leg back to the floor. Do the same thing with your other leg. Next use both legs together. Continue to alternate until you do 10 of each. Work up to 3 sets of 10.

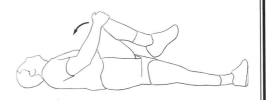

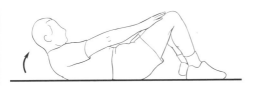

Partial Sit-up

Lie on your back with your knees bent. Do a pelvic tilt and reach with both hands toward your knees. Raise your upper body off the ground about one fourth the way to your knees. Slowly lower yourself back to the floor. Work up to 3 sets of 10.

Rotational Sit-up

Lie on your back with your knees bent. Do a pelvic tilt and then slightly twist as you raise yourself up. Reach with both hands to the outside of one knee. Alternate from side to side. Exhale as you raise yourself up. Work up to 3 sets of 10.

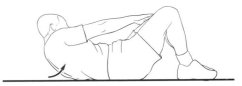

Back Strengthening Exercises

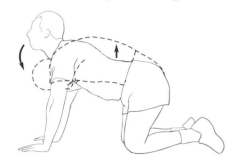

Cat Back Stretch

Kneel on your hands and knees in a relaxed position. Raise your back up like a cat and hold for 5 seconds. Repeat 10 times.

Cobra Stretch

Crouch on your hands and knees. First rock forward onto your extended arms, allowing your back to sag with your head up. Hold for 5 seconds. Then rock back and sit on your bent knees with your arms extended and your head tucked in. Hold for 5 seconds. Repeat 10 times.

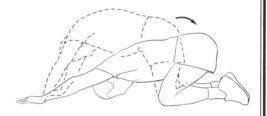

Neck Strengthening Exercises

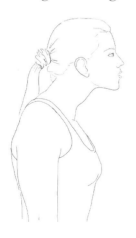

Chin Retractions

Sit in a chair or stand with your weight evenly distributed. Pull your chin toward your throat, sliding your head straight backward. Do not move your head up or down. Hold for 5 seconds. Relax and repeat three times, two to three times daily.

Neck Range-of-Motion Exercises

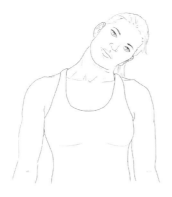
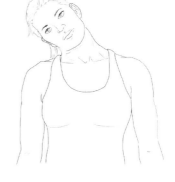
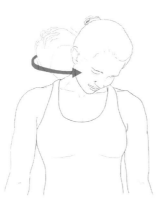
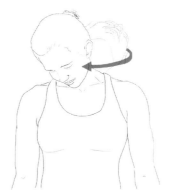

Head Rolls

Sit in a chair or stand with your weight evenly distributed. Begin by gently bowing your head toward your chest, stretching your right ear toward your right shoulder, then your left ear toward your left shoulder. Next, gently roll your head in a circle clockwise three times. Switch directions and gently roll your head in a circle counterclockwise three times.

SHOULDER

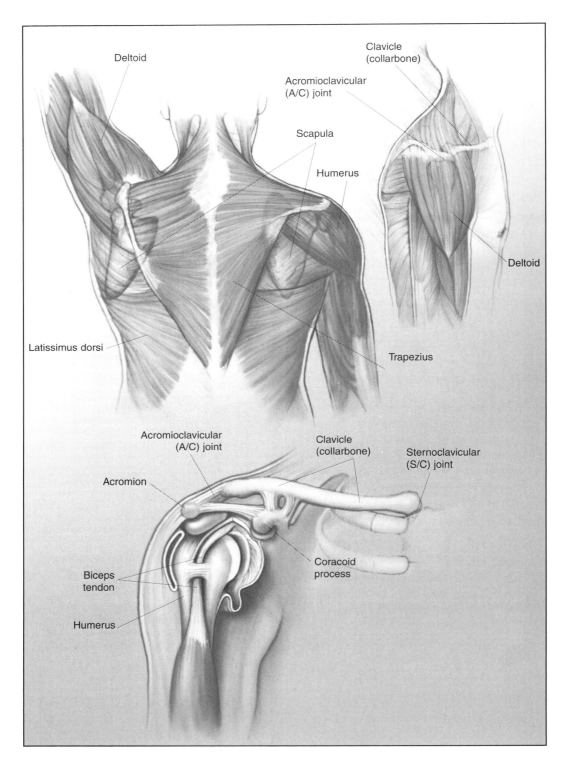

SHOULDER

PICTURE A BASEBALL player as he winds up and fires a ball across home plate at 90 miles per hour. This is one of many images that convey the range of motion and power of the shoulder, the most moveable joint in the body.

It consists of three bones: the collarbone (clavicle), the shoulder blade (scapula), and the upper arm bone (humerus). You may think of the shoulder as having just one joint, where the ball at the end of the arm bone fits into the socket of the shoulder blade (glenohumeral joint). But there is a second one called the acromioclavicular (AC) joint located between the collarbone and the acromion, the part of the shoulder blade that forms the highest part of the shoulder.

A network of strong muscles, tendons, and ligaments hold the shoulder in place. One key part of this network is the rotator cuff—composed of the tendons and muscles situated on top of the shoulder joint to provide strength and support. Other shoulder muscles support the neck, head, and back and make it possible for us to lift heavy objects.

The shoulder's ability to move so freely is also the reason it is vulnerable to injury. Because the ball in the joint is bigger than the socket that holds it, it's easy for the ball to slip out of place even with the strong tissues that surround and support it. Nearly six million people a year see a doctor for a sprain, strain, dislocation, or other shoulder problem.

Athletes account for many of those doctor visits but so do those people who garden, wash windows, or perform other chores that involve overhead arm motions. As we get older and the joint starts to suffer from wear and tear, shoulder pain is also common.

Most shoulder problems can be successfully treated with simple measures such as rest or immobilization in a sling. The most important thing people can do to avoid shoulder problems is this: at the first sign of pain, stop the activity that is aggravating your shoulder. Otherwise, little problems can become big ones.

FROZEN SHOULDER

What It Is

? A person with what's called frozen shoulder doesn't literally wake up one morning with a shoulder that doesn't move. Known by the medical term adhesive capsulitis, a frozen shoulder refers to a gradual loss of range of shoulder motion. Although the cause is unknown, it occurs when an inflammation leads to a tightening of the space between the capsule and ball of the arm bone (humerus) where it fits into the shoulder joint. The tightness and stiffness make even simple arm movements difficult.

Frozen shoulder usually affects people between the ages of 40 and 60. Those with diabetes are at greater risk. If a person with diabetes has a frozen shoulder, nearly half the time both shoulders will be affected. Other people at risk for this condition are those with Parkinson's disease, hyperthyroidism, and cardiovascular disease. A patient whose arm has been immobile for a period of time due to pain from a traumatic injury or shoulder surgery can have the symptoms of frozen shoulder, too.

Signs and Symptoms

At its worst point, you will be able to move your arm only half as far as normal. The pain will be greatest when you move your arm to the limit of its range.

A frozen shoulder typically progresses through stages. First is the "freezing" phase in which pain and stiffness build gradually and cause progressive loss of motion. Eventually, the pain diminishes and moving the arm becomes more comfortable but still limited in the distance it can move. This is what some doctors call the "thawing" phase. Finally, range of motion returns but not always to the same level as before. The whole process can take 6 months or more than 2 years.

When to Call the Doctor

Call if you have these symptoms so the doctor can eliminate other causes and recommend a treatment program that will get you on the road to recovery faster. Also, see your doctor if your shoulder seems stiff, and you are about to start an exercise program so the doctor can look for any internal injury in the shoulder that might be aggravated by excessive movement.

88

How to Treat It

Taking an anti-inflammatory medication such as ibuprofen can help relieve pain. Moist heat followed by gentle exercises three to four times a day should help restore the shoulder's range of motion. Depending on the severity of the pain, the doctor may also recommend a corticosteroid injection into the joint or prescribe muscle relaxants. If after several months your shoulder has shown no improvement, arthroscopic surgery may be recommended. In this type of surgery, the doctor inserts pencil-sized instruments through a tiny incision and is guided by a small fiber optic camera that can project images from inside the body onto a video screen.

Prevention

There aren't really any measures to prevent this condition, but if you seek treatment as soon you notice loss of motion and stiffness, you may be able to limit the severity of the symptoms.

ROTATOR CUFF TEARS

What It Is

A common cause of shoulder pain, especially in the over-40 set, is a rotator cuff tear. The rotator cuff is the network of four muscles and several tendons that form a covering around the top of the upper arm bone (humerus) to hold it in place in the shoulder joint and enable the arm to rotate (see figure).

Although the rotator cuff can be torn from a single traumatic injury, most tears are the result of overuse of these muscles and tendons over a period of years. People who are especially at risk for overuse are those who engage in repetitive overhead motions.

These include participants in sports such as baseball, tennis, weight lifting, and rowing. Occupations that make people vulnerable include house painting and jobs involving heavy lifting.

Most older people who have rotator cuff tears don't have any symptoms, or the symptoms are mild and not disabling. But for those who do have symptoms, the pain and limited range of motion can be quite debilitating.

A rotator cuff tear can be partial or complete, in which the cuff is torn fully through the tissue, and it is usually in the tendon part of the rotator cuff. The latter type of

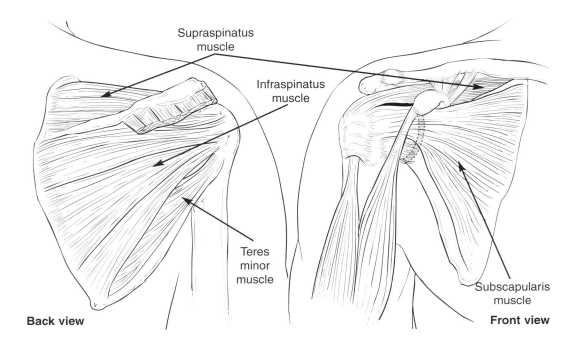

Supraspinatus muscle

Infraspinatus muscle

Teres minor muscle

Subscapularis muscle

Back view

Front view

tear, called a full-thickness tear, is much less common than a partial tear and requires surgery to repair.

Signs and Symptoms

Recurrent shoulder pain is the main symptom. The pain will be especially noticeable when you lift your arm, such as when you are getting dressed. Often you'll have pain at night and difficulty sleeping on the affected side. It's also common to feel weakness or a catching sensation and hear cracking sounds when you lift your arm. Unless it has been triggered by a specific injury, a rotator cuff tear usually occurs in the dominant arm (right side if you are right-handed) since that's the one that gets the most use—or overuse.

When to Call the Doctor

If you have these symptoms for a few days, it's wise to have your shoulder examined by your doctor who will prescribe a treatment regimen based on your specific case.

Diagnostic tests may include MRI (magnetic resonance imaging), which can detect a full tear and can also help to detect a partial one.

How to Treat It

 Your treatment may include one or more of the following

1. Anti-inflammatory medications to ease the pain

2. Applying cold and heat

3. Use of a sling to immobilize the shoulder while it heals

4. Strengthening and stretching exercises under the supervision of a physical therapist

5. Ultrasound treatments

6. Corticosteroid injections

The injections are used for pain relief and to decrease the inflammation but shouldn't be repeated frequently because they can weaken tendons.

If the tear doesn't respond to these treatments or if it is completely through the tissue, surgery is needed to repair the tendon. Following surgery, you'll need to perform exercises to strengthen the muscles and restore range of motion. It may take 6 months or more for the shoulder to return to normal, depending on how diligently you follow the recommended rehabilitation program.

Prevention

Avoid repetitive activities with the arm at shoulder level or higher, especially if they cause pain. If you can't avoid them, you may be able to adjust how you carry them out so you put less strain on your shoulder.

SHOULDER ARTHRITIS

What It Is

Every time you slip into a shirt or comb your hair, your shoulder joint has to move. Multiply those and other daily activities over several decades, and you can understand how your shoulder joints might suffer from all that wear and tear. If the joints become inflamed, it may be due to osteoarthritis (OA), a condition common in people over 50. It's also sometimes referred to as degenerative arthritis.

What happens is that the constant movement of the shoulder over many years can cause the cushion of cartilage between the bones to literally wear away. At that point, the bones start to rub together and the resulting friction irritates the tissue around the bones.

A second, less common type is rheumatoid arthritis (RA), an autoimmune disease that can affect multiple joints in the body and produce symptoms similar to

OA. It usually starts at younger ages than OA, usually after age 30, and women are three times more likely to have it than men.

A third type is posttraumatic arthritis which develops, sometimes years later, after the shoulder has been dislocated or fractured and doesn't heal completely.

People who play sports such as tennis or baseball or whose jobs require vigorous arm movement are especially vulnerable.

Signs and Symptoms

The primary symptom is deep-seated pain that progressively worsens. The pain may be worse in the front or the back of the shoulder, depending on which of the two shoulder joints is affected. If you have RA, both joints can be affected so the pain may be felt in front and back.

Initially, your shoulder may only hurt after you've been involved in strenuous activity. But gradually,

Shoulder Replacement Surgery

Although shoulder joint replacement surgery is less common than knee or hip replacement, it is very successful in reducing pain and restoring range of motion when arthritis symptoms become severe. The procedure works well, not only for older people but also is recommended for those in the 30- to 50-age range, particularly in those patients with RA.

Depending on your particular shoulder problem, the joint may either be repaired or replaced with a prosthesis (artificial joint). The procedure usually requires a hospital stay of 2 to 3 days. You may be given a general or regional anesthetic and have a 3" to 4" incision on the front of your shoulder. Your physical therapy can usually begin the next day. When you return home, you'll need to wear a sling at night for at least a month and avoid certain motions such as pushing yourself up in bed or lifting anything heavier than a coffee cup. You'll also need to diligently follow a program of home exercises to get your shoulder back in peak condition.

It's easy to overwork the shoulder after surgery because you are finally freed from the pain. It's important, though, to follow the doctor's orders about not overdoing it. Otherwise you may damage your shoulder and severely limit your range of motion. For 6 months after the surgery, you should avoid contact sports or heavy lifting.

anytime you move your shoulder it hurts, and it may ache even when it's resting. It may also keep you from getting a good night's sleep. Some people with arthritis may feel a grating or crackling sensation in the shoulder when they move. Others say they can detect a change in the weather, specifically the barometric pressure and higher humidity, because the shoulder aches more.

Arthritis affects your range of motion, too. Because it hurts, you start to favor your shoulder and stop moving it as much. This can lead to stiffening of the muscles and other tissues, thus reducing your flexibility. Combing your hair, for example, or reaching over your head can become difficult.

How to Treat It

Mild pain from OA and posttraumatic arthritis can be treated with an anti-inflammatory medication such as ibuprofen. You also should give your shoulder a rest from activities that aggravate the pain. Ice can help, too, by reducing the inflammation. Apply an ice pack 20 to 30 minutes two or three times a day. Some people may get more relief by using heat. Apply a heating pad, turned to a low setting, for 20 to 40 minutes two or three times a day. Treatment of RA is more complicated and needs to be directed by a physician.

When to Call the Doctor

If you've tried home treatment for a couple of weeks without relief, see your doctor to find out what type of arthritis you have and what additional treatments can be tried to give you pain relief. An X-ray will show whether the joint space has narrowed as a result of the worn out cartilage. It will also show if any bone spurs have developed as a result.

The doctor may prescribe additional medications and physical therapy, since gentle exercises can help restore muscle flexibility and range of motion.

If you are diagnosed with RA, the doctor may recommend corticosteroid injections into the shoulder to relieve pain and can also prescribe drugs used to treat this condition.

In most cases, the symptoms of arthritis can be treated with the measures described above. In stubborn cases where pain persists, surgery can relieve it.

Prevention

Prompt treatment of shoulder injuries, such as fractures and dislocations, may help head off posttraumatic arthritis.

SHOULDER DISLOCATIONS AND INSTABILITY

What It Is

? The shoulder is the most moveable joint in the body, but it's also the most frequently dislocated. Here's why: the shoulder's wide range of motion is possible because of the way the shoulder joint is built—with a shallow cup (glenoid) where the ball at the end of the arm bone (humerus) fits in. But because this cup doesn't provide a deep socket to cradle the ball, the shoulder joint is easily dislocated.

Dislocations occur when the shoulder receives a strong force that pulls the arm in an extreme direction, during a fall or a sports injury, for example. The shoulder joint can dislocate forward, backward, or downward. A common type is a forward slip, where the upper arm bone is forced out of the front part of the joint. (See p 100 on Shoulder Separation.)

The dislocation can be partial, in that the ball is only partly out of the socket, or it can be complete. Usually the force that causes the dislocation also tears ligaments and tendons.

Instability is the word used to describe shoulders that are loose and slip out of place repeatedly. After a dislocation, the capsule or covering of the shoulder joint can remain loose and allow repeated episodes. These may not be as painful as the first time, but they can still be unpleasant.

Signs and Symptoms

With a dislocation, you'll feel intense pain and your shoulder will look out of place (see figure). Pain also is frequently caused by accompanying muscle spasms around the joint. You're also likely to notice bruises, swelling, numbness, and a feeling of weakness.

If the dislocation is not your first, you may feel the shoulder slip and your arm will hurt when you lift it. Some people with shoulder instability describe a feeling that isn't really painful so much as uncomfortable, as if the arm is "dead."

When to Call the Doctor

Go to the hospital emergency room as soon as possible if you think you've dislocated your shoulder. If this is a repeat episode, you aren't in severe pain, and you can soon move your shoulder almost normally, call your doctor for an appointment.

How to Treat It

First the doctor will order X-rays of the shoulder to evaluate the extent of the dislocation and rule out a related fracture. Then you'll be sedated so the doctor can push the shoulder joint back in place—a procedure called a shoulder reduction. Right away the severe pain will be relieved.

Afterward, you'll need to give your shoulder a rest for a few weeks and wear a sling to help keep it from moving. To relieve the soreness and swelling, you can apply ice for 20 to 30 minutes three or four times a day. You'll also need to follow an exercise program to rehabilitate the shoulder. First, you'll start with stretching exercises to return your normal range of motion. Then you can perform strengthening exercises, including use of weights, to build up your muscles to peak condition. This increased strength can help prevent dislocations in the future.

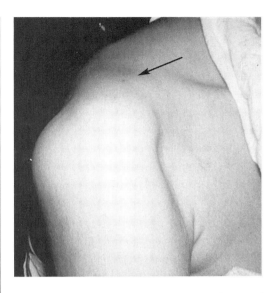

A shoulder that has dislocated once is vulnerable to repeat episodes, especially in young, active people. If you have repeated dislocations due to instability, surgery may be necessary to repair torn or stretched ligaments so they are better able to hold the joint in place. After surgery, you'll need to keep the shoulder immobilized for a few weeks, usually with a sling. Full recovery will require several months of rehabilitation, including 2 to 4 weeks of physical therapy.

Prevention

There is a lot you can do to prevent falls. (See p 38 for some tips.) If you play sports such as football, always wear shoulder pads.

Shoulder Fracture

What It Is

A severe blow to the shoulder can cause a partial or complete crack in a bone. The most common site of a break is the collarbone (clavicle), especially among children and athletes. Because a child's clavicle doesn't completely harden until adulthood, it doesn't take much force to break it. When an athlete fractures this bone, it's sometimes due to a fall on the arm or shoulder, with the force transmitting upward to the bone.

Fractures can sometimes occur at the head or neck of the arm bone (humerus), where it connects the arm to the shoulder. This type of fracture is particularly common in the elderly who have osteoporosis (weak bones).

Fractures of the shoulder blade (scapula) are rare but can occur due to severe trauma from a direct blow such as from a traffic accident or a fall from a significant height.

Signs and Symptoms

You are likely to have severe pain and won't be able to lift your arm. If you do raise it, you may have a grinding sensation due to the broken bone parts rubbing together. In a short time, you may notice bruising or redness, and the shoulder may look deformed or have a bump over the site of the fracture. A broken clavicle can make the shoulder look as if it is sagging.

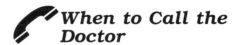

When to Call the Doctor

If you think you've broken your shoulder, head for the hospital emergency room so a doctor can X-ray it and determine the site and severity of the break.

How to Treat It

Most shoulder fractures can be treated with a sling for a few weeks. An anti-inflammatory medication such as ibuprofen can help control the accompanying pain and inflammation.

A broken clavicle in a child may heal in 3 to 4 weeks, while an adult many need 4 to 6 weeks to recover. A couple of weeks or so after the injury, you can usually begin gentle range-of-motion exercises, assuming your pain has significantly diminished. A large bump may develop where the break occurred, but this will likely shrink over time but may never completely disappear. The younger the person, the more likely the bone will return to a normal appearance.

In the case of other types of breaks, your doctor will advise you on how long to wear the sling, when to begin gentle exercises, and how to perform them.

Only in rare cases is surgery needed to fix a shoulder fracture, depending on its location, how much the bone has been pushed out of place, and whether soft tissues such as ligaments are also damaged. After surgery, the shoulder will be immobilized until the bone heals enough that you can begin moving it. Since each

Throwing Injuries

Overuse of the shoulder, such as repeated overhead throwing, can cause microscopic cracks (or stress fractures) in the head of the humerus where it fits into the shoulder joint. In children, this is called Little Leaguer's shoulder. The condition is sometimes seen in swimmers, too. Stress fractures, also called fatigue fractures, cause a gradual onset of pain. Any persistent pain, weakness, or loss of motion should disqualify a child from playing until these findings resolve or are evaluated by a physician.

Pitching Recommendations for Young Baseball Players

Age	Maximum Pitches Per Game	Maximum Games Per Week
8-10	52 ± 15	2 ± 0.6
11-12	68 ± 18	2 ± 0.6
13-14	76 ± 16	2 ± 0.4
15-16	91 ± 16	2 ± 0.6
17-18	106 ± 16	2 ± 0.6

Because it is hard to distinguish this injury from other causes of shoulder pain, it's wise to see a doctor for a diagnosis. Sometimes a bone scan is necessary to determine whether the bone is cracked. This condition can usually be treated by simply giving the shoulder a rest from the activity that is causing it. This allows the bone time to regenerate and repair the cracks.

case varies depending on the severity and location of the break, your doctor will advise you on the physical therapy you'll need and the length of time your rehabilitation will take.

Prevention

✔ Shoulder pads offer protection during activities in which a fall on the shoulder might occur such as football, dirt bike riding, and snowboarding, for example.

SHOULDER PAIN

What It Is

? A day spent hanging wallpaper or playing some serious tennis after a long layoff can leave you with a sore shoulder. Take this as a sign to give your shoulder a rest. It's easy to ignore a little mild aching and keep up your pace, but working through the pain can lead to more serious problems, especially as you get older. Some people ignore mild symptoms for months before seeking treatment.

Overuse can cause a condition called impingement syndrome. Impingement refers to excessive rubbing or squeezing in the shoulder joint and rotator cuff (tendons and muscles surrounding the joint). One or a combination of conditions may cause this, including bursitis, tendinitis, or even a torn rotator cuff. The rubbing or pinching may occur as a result of a bony spur that puts pressure on or repeatedly rubs the tendon. The squeezing occurs

because the tissues have become irritated and swollen with too much use.

People with jobs that give their arms and shoulders a workout, house painters, wallpaper hangers, and electricians for example, are especially vulnerable.

Bursitis is an inflammation of the lubricating sac (bursa) located just over the rotator cuff. Bursitis is caused by frequently extending your arm such as happens when you pitch a baseball, paint a wall, or wash your windows. If you don't give the shoulder time to heal, the symptoms can become progressively worse.

Tendinitis is an inflammation of the shoulder tendons that develops over time. Older people sometimes will have this condition if they jump into a heavy-duty training program without having conditioned their muscles first.

Signs and Symptoms

With impingement, you may notice only minor pain and a slight loss of strength in your arm, and you may not be able to lift your arm as high as you normally could because that makes the pain worse. The pain may be centered in the upper shoulder or the upper part of the arm. It's also common for your shoulder to ache at night and can keep you from getting enough sleep.

With bursitis, the pain can range from mild to severe and your movement will be limited. A sign of tendinitis is an inability to hold the arm in certain positions. Repeated episodes of tendinitis could indicate a torn rotator cuff. (See p 89 for more information.)

How to Treat It

Fortunately, these conditions usually can be treated easily if you begin promptly. The main treatment is resting the shoulder. An ice pack applied for 20 to 30 minutes two or three times a day will help reduce pain and swelling. An anti-inflammatory medication such as ibuprofen can make you more comfortable. Don't resume vigorous activities using your arm and shoulder until the pain is gone.

When to Call the Doctor

If the pain is acute or if it persists after you've tried treating it yourself, call your doctor. Call, too, if you have repeated episodes. You may be advised to wear a sling, take prescription medications, or begin a physical therapy program that includes ultrasound therapy—gentle sound vibrations that warm deep tissue to improve blood flow. Sometimes corticosteroid injections are used to relieve the symptoms.

Once the pain subsides, your doctor will recommend a series of exercises to restore the shoulder's flexibility and strength. It's a good idea to apply heat before beginning stretching exercises. Heat loosens up the muscles and can be applied by taking a hot shower, soaking in a hot bath, or using a moist-heat heating pad.

In a few cases, the damage may be so extensive that surgery is required to repair the shoulder. The operation takes about an hour and can usually be done arthroscopically (using pencil-sized instruments through a small incision and guided by a tiny fiber optic camera). Less than half of patients have to stay in the hospital overnight. You'll need to wear a shoulder immobilizer or sling for about 2 to 3 weeks and limit how much you move your arm. Physical therapy restores strength and range of motion. Most people are pain-free within 4 to 6 weeks.

Prevention

 Don't "work through" pain! If you feel discomfort, give the shoulder a rest.

SHOULDER SEPARATION

What It Is

Take a tumble off a bicycle and you could share a common ailment with a host of football quarterbacks—a separated shoulder. The injury typically occurs from a sharp blow to the tip of your shoulder, which causes a separation where the collarbone (clavicle) connects to the shoulder blade (scapula) at the acromioclavicular (AC) joint.

The damage actually occurs to one or both of the main ligaments that hold the two bones together. If either is partially or completely torn, the end of the clavicle can slip out of place. The severity of the injury can vary greatly from a mild separation caused by a sprain to the AC ligament to complete tears of both ligaments.

Signs and Symptoms

Just as the extent of the injury varies, so do the symptoms. A mild sprain can cause the area over the AC joint to be tender, which makes

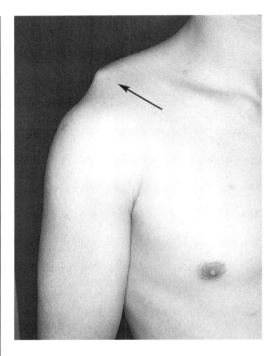

lifting your arm somewhat painful. If both ligaments tear, you will not only have more severe pain, but you will probably notice that the shoulder appears deformed. You might see a bump at the tip of the shoulder where the AC joint is located (see arrow on figure).

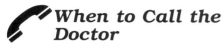

When to Call the Doctor

If the pain persists and if you notice a bump, see your doctor. If you have severe pain and your shoulder looks deformed, head to the hospital emergency room.

How to Treat It

Your doctor may X-ray your shoulder while you hold a light weight to make the separation more pronounced and therefore more visible on the film. An X-ray of your uninjured shoulder also might be taken for purposes of comparison.

If the separation is mild, you will probably just wear a sling to immobilize your shoulder for a few days until the pain goes away. Icing your shoulder during the first 48 hours will help reduce the swelling and pain. Use an ice pack for 20 to 30 minutes, two or three times a day. You can also take an anti-inflammatory medication such as ibuprofen for pain relief. As the swelling decreases, the bones may settle back into place within the joint.

After the initial treatment, you'll be advised to perform exercises to restore your range of motion. In cases of mild sprains, you may be able to return to normal activities and sports within a month. More serious dislocations take longer to heal. Your doctor may recommend physical therapy to help the healing process.

If both ligaments are torn, you may need surgery to repair them. Following surgery, you'll have to wear a sling for about a month and undergo physical therapy for 2 to 4 weeks.

ELBOW AND FOREARM

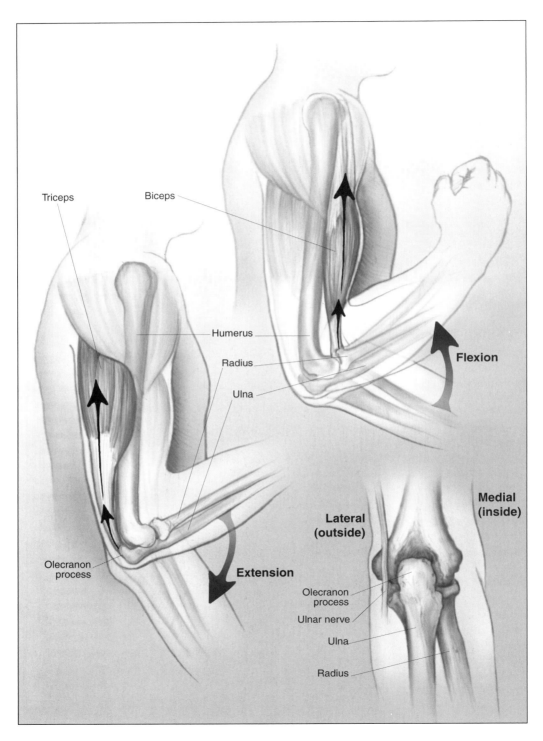

Triceps

Biceps

Humerus

Radius

Ulna

Flexion

Lateral
(outside)

Medial
(inside)

Olecranon
process

Extension

Olecranon
process

Ulnar nerve

Ulna

Radius

ELBOW AND FOREARM

Without your elbow, your arm would be a pretty useless appendage. One of the body's most important hinge joints, the elbow is formed when the humerus, the bone in your upper arm, links up with the two smaller bones, the radius and the ulna, that run through the forearm from the elbow to the hand. The radius can rotate over the ulna, allowing you to hold your arm straight out and rotate the palm of your hand.

The elbow can't bend on its own, of course. That's where the muscles come in. If you contract the biceps on the front of the upper arm, the elbow bends. If you contract the triceps muscles, on the back of the upper arm, the elbow extends.

So where does the funny bone (also known as the crazy bone) come in? Actually, it's not really a bone but rather a projection or knobby bump on the side of the elbow called the olecranon. The ulnar nerve passes through a groove in it and since there's only skin covering the area, a sharp rap on it puts pressure on the nerve and sends a sharp tingling pain down your arm to your fingers. The name "funny bone" probably derives from the odd feeling this causes, but most people would say the momentary pain isn't funny at all!

DISLOCATED ELBOW

What It Is

The natural response when you feel yourself falling is to stretch out your hand to break the fall. Unfortunately, the impact can knock the bones in your elbow out of position.

Signs and Symptoms

If you dislocate your elbow, you'll know it. You'll feel intense pain, and you won't be able to bend your elbow. It will also begin to swell and will look deformed.

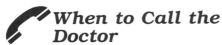

When to Call the Doctor

Try to immobilize the arm and then seek medical help immediately. To immobilize it, make a splint by wrapping a folded blanket, pillow, or folded newspapers around the elbow.

How to Treat It

Once you get to the hospital emergency room, a physician will gently manipulate the bones back in place after administering either a local anesthetic or conscious sedation. With con-

Elbows or Fingers?

In children, the elbow is the most commonly dislocated joint. But in adults, shoulder and finger dislocations happen more often.

scious sedation, you're given a drug intravenously that makes you drowsy. It also has an amnesia effect so you don't remember the procedure. If a few hours pass between the time of your injury and when it's treated, you may need a general anesthesia before manipulation because swelling and muscle spasms will have worsened, making the procedure itself very painful.

Once your elbow is back in place, the doctor will probably order X-rays to make sure there were no fractures or other damage. If a fracture is found, additional treatment may be necessary. (See p 111 for details on fracture treatment.)

If the elbow was merely dislocated and no fracture was found, you'll be told to wear a splint for a few weeks. Anti-inflammatory drugs such as ibuprofen can help with pain relief. When your doctor decides the elbow has healed sufficiently, you can start exercising, with the help of a physical therapist, so the joint can return to full function.

Prevention

There are lots of things you can do to prevent falls. (See p 38 for tips on fall prevention.)

ELBOW ARTHRITIS

What It Is

? Arthritis in the elbow is an inflammation of the joint that results in pain and swelling. One common cause is rheumatoid arthritis (RA), a disease of the joint linings. The lining swells, the joint space narrows, and gradually the disease destroys bone and soft tissue (see figure, left, below). Usually, you'll have RA in both elbows and also in other joints such as the hand, wrist and shoulder.

Another type of arthritis is osteoarthritis, also called OA or "wear-and-tear" arthritis, in which the cushioning cartilage at the ends of the bones deteriorates, and the bones begin to rub together. This sometimes happens with repetitive use, such as with baseball pitchers or certain types of manual laborers. This can cause fragments of bone and cartilage—also called loose bodies—to break away and act like gravel to wear down the joint (see figure, right, below). OA is less common in the elbow than it is in weight-bearing joints such as the hip or the knee.

Elbow arthritis may also result from an injury that damages the cartilage. This is called post-traumatic arthritis.

Signs and Symptoms

The common signs of RA are pain and swelling. In the early stages, the pain usually cen-

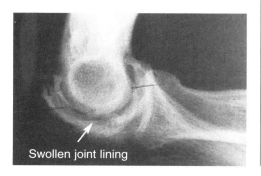

Swollen joint lining

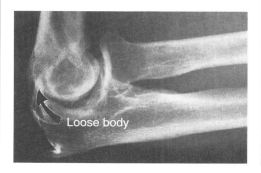

Loose body

ters on the outside of the elbow and is most noticeable when you turn or rotate your straightened arm. In later stages, the pain worsens and the elbow becomes unstable, meaning that the ligaments soften and therefore don't contain the elbow joint as firmly as they should.

With OA, the pain intensifies as you bend your elbow, and it may be noticeable at night as well as during the day even when your elbow is at rest. If there are loose bodies in the elbow, they can become "trapped" between joint surfaces and limit range of motion in the elbow.

Gradually, the pain and limited mobility of an arthritic elbow make even light household or office tasks difficult.

How Do I Know I Have Arthritis?

1. *An inability to straighten or bend the elbow*

2. *Catching" or locking, particularly with OA, if there are loose bodies in the elbow*

3. *Stiffness, especially with post-traumatic arthritis, particularly when you first get up in the morning*

4. *Warmth or redness around the joint*

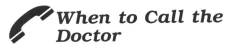

When to Call the Doctor

Swelling, stiffness, and pain in the elbow joint could be a sign of arthritis but could also be caused by other conditions that are easily treatable. If you've tried home remedies for a few weeks (resting the elbow, applying ice, and taking an anti-inflammatory medication) but the symptoms persist, you should call your doctor.

How to Treat It

You and your doctor can discuss an array of treatments both medical and physical that will work best for your particular type of arthritis. For example, if you have arthritis caused by overuse, modifying your sports or job activities can help relieve symptoms. So can applying heat and cold and performing gentle exercises. Various medications are used for pain relief. Sometimes a splint that allows movement but also protects the elbow from stress is helpful.

When other measures offer little or no relief, your doctor may recommend surgical options that can reduce pain and increase your range of motion. These can run the gamut from arthroscopy, which uses pencil-sized instruments and a fiber optic camera to make two or more tiny incisions, to arthroplasty, in which the surgeon creates an artificial joint.

Prevention

✔ Scientists have not yet determined how to prevent RA. You may be able to head off the effects of OA by limit-ing activities in which there is repetitive use. It's also important that you seek treatment promptly if you sustain trauma to the elbow.

ELBOW BURSITIS

What It Is

? Because your elbow sticks out from your body when your arm is slightly bent, it's an easy target for getting banged on doorjambs, walls, and all manner of things. If you bump your elbow and it becomes painful or swollen, that's a sign of bursitis. But bursitis can be pain-less, too, and be noticeable only because of localized swelling at the tip of the elbow. This swelling can range from the size of a pea to larger than a baseball.

Technically, what you have is an inflammation of the bursa, a slip-pery sac beneath the skin of the elbow. The bursa is there to act as a cushion between the skin and the bone. But if you bang your elbow against a hard surface or press on it too long, the bursa becomes irritated. People in cer-tain occupations are especially vulnerable, particularly plumbers or heating and air conditioning technicians who have to crawl on their knees into tight spaces and lean on their elbows. People who

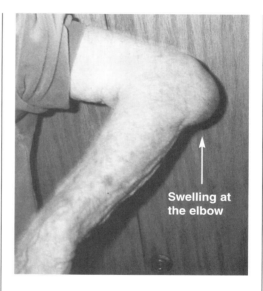

Swelling at the elbow

have to bend their elbows fre-quently, such as painters, are also at risk.

Signs and Symptoms

If your elbow swells sudden-ly, it's probably because it suffered a blow. The skin may be scraped or cut, too. If the swelling is gradual, it is more likely due to a long-lasting condi-tion such as pressure from leaning on something. As the swelling goes down, there may be a lump at the end of the elbow.

The elbow may be painful or just tender to touch, and you may not be able to move it as much as you normally do. If the skin is red or hot, you could have an infection. The swelling can become so large that it's hard to put on a long-sleeve shirt.

How to Treat It

If the swelling developed gradually and isn't very large, try RICE (Rest, Ice, Compression, Elevation) at home.

1. Stop doing activities that put pressure on the elbow.

2. Use an ice pack for 15 to 20 minutes, three or four times a day.

3. Wrap an elastic bandage around the elbow to reduce the swelling.

4. Raise the elbow above the level of your heart.

When to Call the Doctor

If the symptoms persist after you've tried the RICE method, or if your elbow looks red at the location of the swelling and the pain increases, call your doctor. You should also call if the swelling developed suddenly as the result of a direct blow to the elbow, because you may need an X-ray to determine if it's fractured.

Sometimes, doctors recommend aspirating (removing the fluid from) the bursa with a syringe to reduce the pain and swelling. Taking anti-inflammatory medications such as ibuprofen can also help. Or, the doctor may inject a powerful anti-inflammatory drug, a corticosteroid, to heal the bursa. If the symptoms are chronic or recurring, the doctor may recommend surgically removing the bursa.

Prevention

Bursitis is difficult to prevent, particularly if you work in one of the professions listed above.

ELBOW FRACTURES

What It Is

 The knobby bone that sticks out from under the skin covering your elbow is called the olecranon. There isn't much in the way of tissue to cushion and protect it, so the bone can break if it takes a direct blow or if you fall on your bent elbow.

Signs and Symptoms

A fracture will cause immediate and intense pain. There will likely be bruising and swelling, and if the bone also is dislocated, the elbow may look odd or out of alignment. One or more of your fingers may be numb, too.

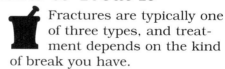 When to Call the Doctor

Contact your doctor immediately. An X-ray of the bone will reveal the type of fracture you have and therefore what treatment is required. The doctor will also look for any possible damage to blood vessels or nerves.

How to Treat It

Fractures are typically one of three types, and treatment depends on the kind of break you have.

In a type I fracture, the bone hasn't moved out of place very much. Usually this can be treated with a splint or sling that holds the elbow at a 90-degree angle. Some gentle hand and wrist exercises performed daily help the healing process.

Type II fractures are the most common. In this type, the bone has separated and the parts are slightly misaligned, so surgery is necessary to pin the bone parts back together. A few weeks of physical therapy after the surgery will help maintain your range of motion.

Sports Injuries to the Elbow

Sometimes athletes sustain stress fractures in elbows. A stress fracture is a tiny crack in the bone caused by repetitive bending and pressure on the elbow joint. Baseball pitchers are prone to it, for example. This type of fracture can be treated initially by resting the injured area and restricting the activity that caused it. Then the athlete is advised to perform special exercises for several weeks. Full recovery can take 3 to 6 months.

In type III fractures, the most serious kind, the bones are more separated than in type II fractures. The broken part may even be sticking out of the skin. This is called an open fracture, and it requires immediate surgery because of the risk of infection. In these cases, the doctor usually attaches a plate to hold the bones in their proper place. The surgery is followed by several weeks of physical therapy.

If just the very tip of the olecranon breaks off but the joint itself isn't fractured, the doctor may simply remove the small bone fragment and repair the nearby tendon.

ELBOW FRACTURES IN CHILDREN

What It Is

? Although elbow fractures account for only about 10% of all the fractures in children, they can be the among the most serious if not treated properly and promptly. Usually the injury is sports related. The child falls on an outstretched arm with enough force that one of the bones breaks.

Signs and Symptoms

A broken elbow is very painful. Swelling is common, and the child will have difficulty moving the elbow. It may look seriously deformed, too (arrow).

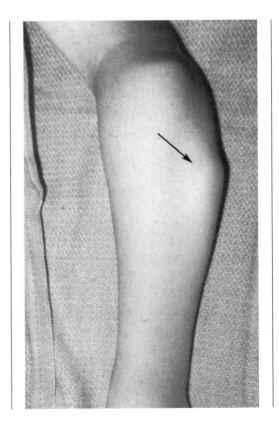

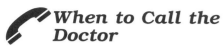

When to Call the Doctor

If the child falls, then complains of pain and refuses to move his elbow, call the doctor or go to the hospital emergency room at once. Even if the pain seems mild, it's wise to have the arm checked out because any kind of damage can lead to long-term disability without careful treatment.

Occasionally, the fracture affects the growth plate, for example, and growth can be arrested and the elbow become deformed over time.

Typically, an X-ray of the elbow is needed to determine if the bone is broken. The doctor will also examine the arm to detect possible damage to nerves or blood vessels. Since the child's bones are still forming, X-rays of both arms may be needed to make comparisons before reaching a final diagnosis.

How to Treat It

If the bone is not displaced or only slightly displaced, the child may need to wear a cast or a splint for a few weeks, usually 3 to 5. Frequently, though, surgery is required to reposition the bones and stabilize them with pins, screws, or other devices. Following the surgery, the child usually will need to wear a cast for 3 to 6 weeks.

Prevention

Often, certain types of protective equipment, such as elbow guards or pads, are recommended for your children's sports. Insist your kids wear them.

ELBOW PAIN

What It Is

Most people who have "tennis elbow" (technically called epicondylitis) don't even play tennis. It's also a familiar complaint of golfers, baseball pitchers, gardeners, and others who make a repetitive motion with one of their arms. If you spend a weekend at home painting, raking, turning a screwdriver, or hammering, for example, tennis elbow can develop. Any activity that requires rotating the arm and extending the wrist can lead to this condition.

Overusing the arm muscles can cause tiny tears in the tendons that attach the muscles in your forearms to your elbow. If you don't give those tears time to heal, the tendon becomes painful. Tennis elbow usually affects adults between 35 and 50 years, with the peak years being the 40s.

Signs and Symptoms

In tennis elbow, the pain develops gradually and is centered around the knobby bump (olecranon) on the outside of the elbow. Golfers and handball players more commonly feel the pain on the inside knob, the part of the elbow that's closest to the body. If your pain is on the inside, you may be told you have "golfer's elbow."

The discomfort may radiate down your forearm. Gripping or lifting something can make the pain worse. In a few cases, the pain starts as a result of a direct blow to the elbow that causes some damage to the muscle and leads to pain when you engage in activities that cause the elbow to move a lot.

How to Treat It

The simple solution is to stop doing whatever it is that caused the symptoms and give your tendons time to heal. Take anti-inflammatory drugs such as ibuprofen to relieve the pain. Applying ice packs for 10 minutes at a time can help, too. Just don't overdo it on the ice because you can actually get frostbite.

Put That Elbow on Ice

Here's an easy way to ice a tennis elbow. Freeze water in an insulated foam or paper cup. Then you can remove the cup from the freezer, tear down the sides to expose the ice and rub over the elbow while holding the base of the cup. Return the unused portion to the freezer to use again later. Normally, ice should not be applied directly to the skin because of the danger of frostbite. To avoid that problem during ice massage, keep the ice moving a circular motion so it doesn't remain in contact with one spot on the elbow's skin. Limit the ice massage to a few minutes.

When the acute pain subsides, you can try some gentle exercises to strengthen the forearm.

In some cases of tennis elbow, injections of a cortisone-based steroid are given to relieve the discomfort. As an alternative to steroids, acupuncture can be used.

You may need to wear an arm brace until the elbow heals fully, and there are many available that can help decrease the symptoms. Elbow sleeves, for example, support the injured muscle and keep it warm. Straps worn just below the elbow joint encircle the muscle and alter the way the elbow moves until it heals. You can buy arm braces at sporting goods stores or pharmacies. If your doctor prescribes a brace, it may be covered by your insurance.

• •

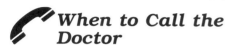

When to Call the Doctor

If the pain hasn't subsided in 3 to 4 weeks or if it becomes worse despite home treatment, call your doctor. Also call if you have other symptoms such as marked weakness or loss of muscle bulk, as these could be signs of neurologic (nervous system) problems.

Prevention

If you noticed the pain after playing a sport, it's a good idea to make sure you are using the right equipment and the right technique. For example, switching to a lighter weight tennis racket may help. Or, if the handle of the racket is too small, wrap it with tape to make it easier to grip.

In bowling, make sure the ball is not too heavy and the finger grip size is appropriate. Consult a reputable sporting goods dealer familiar with your sport for advice on proper equipment fit. If the problem was the result of some other activity such as hammering, take frequent breaks when you resume.

Also, continue with the strengthening exercises as you return to your activity to prevent a recurrence.

LITTLE LEAGUER'S ELBOW

What It Is

? Pitchers on youth baseball teams sometimes pitch too many innings. Or they don't use the proper technique. The result is a painful elbow, sometimes called Little Leaguer's elbow. Shoulders can be affected, too.

Although these may seem like a minor, temporary problem, parents and coaches should take precautions to prevent this injury because the elbows and shoulders of a growing child are still developing. This makes them vulnerable to damage that could become permanent or could at least prevent the child from continuing to play in that sport.

Because this injury happens so frequently, the Little League and other national youth baseball organizations have established rules that limit the number of innings an individual player may pitch, depending on age. For example, Little League limits 12-year-olds to six innings a week. Unfortunately, some children still pitch too much because they play on multiple teams or because coaches don't always enforce limits or they let kids keep playing even when their arms are sore.

Signs and Symptoms

 Repetitive throwing can create too much pull on the tendons and ligaments on the inside of the elbow and too much pressure from compression on the outside. The player will feel pain at the knobby bump (olecranon) on the inside of the elbow. There may be swelling, the elbow's range of motion may be restricted, or the elbow may feel as if it's locking.

How to Treat It

 The pain is sending a message. Your child should stop throwing and let the elbow rest. If your child ignores it, there can be serious complications. The tearing may pull away tiny bone

How Many is Too Many?

Studies show that 20% of children 8 to 12 years of age and 45% of those 13 to 14 will suffer from arm pain during a season of youth baseball. The American Academy of Orthopaedic Surgeons has said a reasonable guideline is for a pitcher to throw a maximum of 80 to 100 pitches during a game or 30 to 40 pitches during a practice. Watch a few practices and talk to the coach about safety measures before you sign your child up for a particular team. As a parent, you should keep track of the number of pitches your young athlete throws in a week. Kids are not likely to keep track, so often it is up to you. Any persistent pain, weakness, or loss of motion should disqualify a child from playing until these findings resolve or are evaluated by a physician.

Pitching Recommendations for Young Baseball Players

Age	Maximum Pitches Per Game	Maximum Games Per Week
8-10	52 ± 15	2 ± 0.6
11-12	68 ± 18	2 ± 0.6
13-14	76 ± 16	2 ± 0.4
15-16	91 ± 16	2 ± 0.6
17-18	106 ± 16	2 ± 0.6

fragments that can disrupt normal growth and cause a permanent deformity. Or your child could sustain a fracture.

You can also apply ice packs 10 to 15 minutes each hour to reduce the swelling.

• •

When to Call the Doctor

If the pain persists despite a few days of complete rest, or if the pain returns when the child resumes pitching, take your child to the doctor for treatment.

Prevention

Aside from limiting the number of throws, coaches can also teach kids proper technique. Youth pitchers often lead with their elbows when they throw, whereas professional ball players lead with their hips, a motion that puts less strain on the elbows. All athletes should warm up their muscles before beginning strenuous play. Regular exercises that strengthen and stretch the arm and shoulder muscles help prevent strains, too.

PULLED ELBOW

What It Is

A common injury to children under 5 years, a pulled elbow is caused by someone pulling sharply on a child's arm causing the ligament to slip between the bones of the joint. Young children are prone to it because their elbow joints are more elastic, and the bones not fully developed compared with that of older children and adults.

It happens for the most innocent reasons. You can be walking hand in hand when the child suddenly decides to run and pulls away from you while you're still tightly clasping his hand. Or maybe you

grab your child's arm to prevent him from running into the street. The next thing you know, your child is crying and can't move his arm. Fortunately, it's a problem that is easily fixed.

Signs and Symptoms

You may hear a popping sound when the elbow dislocates. The child will begin crying in pain immediately, and the arm will hang limp at his side with the elbow bent slightly. The elbow may also appear displaced, as if the bump of the elbow is slightly off to one side. The pain may subside, and the child won't seem to be in much distress except that he won't want to move his arm.

How to Treat It

Take your child to the doctor or hospital emergency room as soon as it happens. If your child is able to bend the arm a bit, a cloth sling to support the elbow and keep it

from moving can make your child more comfortable while you travel to the doctor.

It's a relatively simple procedure to pop the elbow back into place, and it doesn't usually require an anesthetic but it should be done only by someone with medical training. The pain should stop immediately once the elbow is manipulated back to its proper position. Many times it will pop back into place on its own en route to the doctor's office, but you should still have your child examined.

Prevention

Never pull your child up or swing him around by the arms. Explain this to your older children, too, so they won't inadvertently hurt their younger siblings. It's a good idea to caution your caregiver and the child's other relatives such as grandparents, too, in case they aren't aware of risks.

Kids Say the Darnedest Things

Even though the elbow is the source of the problem, your child may say his shoulder hurts, or his collarbone or his wrist. He can't always isolate the source of what's ailing him. But he'll wince if you touch his elbow and that's a good clue that you've located the cause of the trouble

HAND AND WRIST

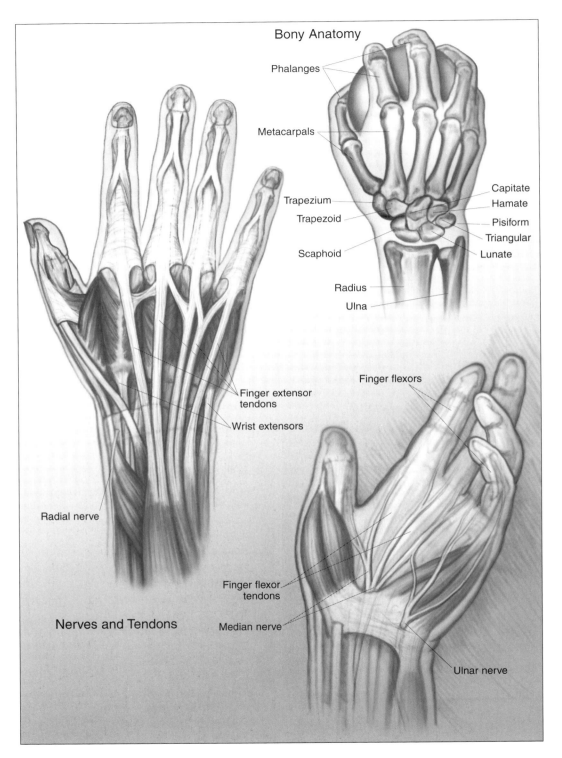

Bony Anatomy

Phalanges

Metacarpals

Capitate
Hamate
Trapezium
Pisiform
Trapezoid
Triangular
Scaphoid
Lunate

Radius

Ulna

Finger flexors

Finger extensor
tendons

Wrist extensors

Radial nerve

Finger flexor
tendons

Nerves and Tendons

Median nerve

Ulnar nerve

HAND AND WRIST

T HE HUMAN HAND IS AN instrument of amazing versatility, delicacy, sensitivity, and strength. It can perform virtually an unlimited variety of tasks, ranging from the delicate (sewing, writing, playing a musical instrument, painting a work of art, bathing a baby, expressing affection with a touch) to the muscular (climbing a rope, sailing a boat, sculpting, doing push-ups, and even delivering a knock-out punch or a karate chop that can break a brick!).

The skeleton of the hand and wrist allows for a combination of great mobility and strength. The eight carpal bones that form the wrist rest on the end of the two bones of the forearm (the radius and ulna). This arrangement allows for a near-universal joint at the wrist. The five metacarpals in the middle part of the hand rest on the eight carpal bones. No less than 14 finger bones, called phalanges, make up the palm. At the ends of the metacarpals are three phalanx bones in each finger, and two in the thumb, with joints in between that allow movement.

Many of the muscles that move the fingers are in the forearm, with long tendons that extend into the hand. This allows for strength from a large muscle mass without bulk in the hand itself. Within the palm of the hand is a additional system of muscles that add further delicacy and versatility of movement. Three important nerves supply sensation to the hand: the ulnar, median, and radial nerves. You may have heard of the median nerve in connection with carpal tunnel syndrome in which swollen tendons put pressure on that nerve, causing numbness in the fingers, wrist pain, and night wakening.

Your hands are the key tools used in most daily activities. Because they are exposed and in contact with the outside world, they can be especially prone to injury. The hand is the most common site of an animal bite, for example, which, because of the risk of infection, can be quite serious. Lacerations can cut nerves, tendons, and blood vessels. Fractures are common. Finger nails also can suffer injury or can become infected through unsanitary manicures.

CARPAL TUNNEL SYNDROME

What It Is

? Carpal tunnel syndrome (CTS) is a condition in which the tendons in the wrist swell and put pressure on the median nerve, one of the three important nerves that supply sensation to the hand. This nerve, surrounded by tendons, passes from the forearm to the hand through the carpal tunnel. Since this tunnel-like structure is narrow, any swelling of the tendons puts pressure on the median nerve and creates the symptoms. Usually, but not always, only one wrist is affected.

There can be many causes of swelling in the wrist tendons. Although the condition can be aggravated by work that involves repetitive grasping of the hands or bending of the wrists, people who don't work with their hands can have CTS, too. CTS is sometimes related to hormonal changes associated with pregnancy and menopause, which helps explain why more women are affected by it than are men. CTS usually goes away when the pregnancy ends. It's also associated with medical conditions such as diabetes, rheumatoid arthritis, and thyroid gland imbalance. Some cases of CTS have no known cause.

Signs and Symptoms

At first, you may feel a painful tingling in your hands, especially at night after using them a lot during the day. The feeling might resemble that of your foot "going to sleep." The pain may even be serious enough to wake you at night. You may have decreased sensation in your thumb and fingers, although not usually the little finger. Some people say it feels as if their fingers are swollen even though they don't appear to be.

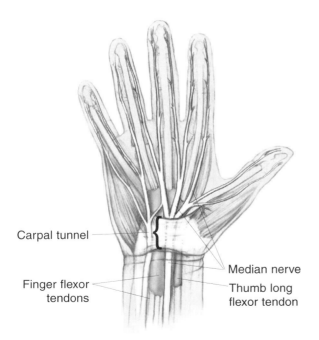

Carpal tunnel

Finger flexor tendons

Median nerve

Thumb long flexor tendon

The pain may radiate up the arm all the way to the shoulder. Manual activity involving your wrist or holding the wrists flexed in one position for long periods such as while driving the car can increase the pain. As you lose sensation in the fingers, you may feel clumsy or have trouble picking up objects, tying your shoes, or twisting lids off of jars. Some people even have trouble distinguishing between hot and cold by touch.

How to Treat It

When you first notice the symptoms, try resting your wrist to reduce the swelling of the tendons and the pressure on the nerve. Commercially available wrist splints can keep the wrist from bending.

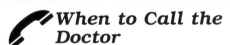

When to Call the Doctor

If the symptoms persist after a few days, see your doctor. Nonsurgical treatments are usually more effective if CTS is diagnosed and treated early. You may be advised to wear hard splints at night and soft ones during the day. Anti-inflammatory drugs such as ibuprofen help reduce swelling and relieve the pain. In some cases, the doctor may recommend a corticosteroid injection in the wrist. A short course of acupuncture also may be effective in relieving symptoms.

Most people respond to such treatments. But, if after about 3 months there is no improvement, outpatient surgery is an option. The surgeon cuts the ligament that forms the roof of the carpal tunnel to make more room and relieve pressure on the nerve. After surgery, you'll notice relief almost immediately although the incision may remain tender until it heals and the stitches are removed. You'll be taught hand and wrist exercises to rebuild circulation, muscle strength, and joint flexibility, and it may be several weeks before you can return to your normal level of physical activities. When you do, it's wise to avoid continuous repetitive movements by alternating activities as much as possible.

Prevention

There are no prevention measures for some of the medical causes of CTS. However, you may be able to prevent some of the repetitive stress your wrist receives, such as when you use a computer keyboard. Try adjusting your work area so that more of your tasks can be performed without bending the wrist up or down. This may be as simple as changing the height of your chair or using a wrist guard with your keyboard.

DUPUYTREN'S DISEASE

What It Is

? A fairly common condition, Dupuytren's disease causes one or more fingers to contract toward the palm of the hand. Although it's not known exactly why, the connective tissue under the skin of the palm begins to thicken and shorten, which is what causes fingers to curl into the palm.

The problem is hereditary and is seven times more likely to affect men than women. It doesn't usually affect people under age 40, although a few children and teens have been known to have an aggressive form of the disease. There's also a higher risk for people who are smokers, diabetics, alcoholics, or those who take anticonvulsant drugs for epilepsy.

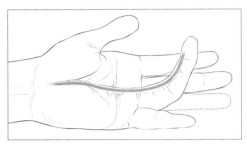

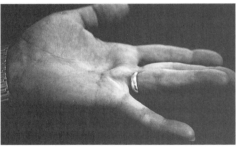

the little and middle fingers, the thumb and the index finger. The progress of the disease is unpredictable.

Signs and Symptoms

The first sign usually is a lump (nodule) in the palm of the hand, often near the base of the ring finger or the little finger. It may look like a callus and it doesn't hurt, although it might be tender if you press on it. As the condition progresses, more lumps appear. Sometimes bands of tough tissue spread into the finger and cause it to curl toward the palm. Typically, the ring finger is affected first, followed by

How to Treat It

Dupuytren's disease isn't painful, and if the nodules don't develop enough to contract the finger, you can ignore them unless they become so large they interfere with your hand function. If the nodules cause contraction of the fingers, you could eventually have trouble putting on gloves or picking up objects, for example. Splints worn at night may slow the progress of the contraction, but surgery to remove the diseased tissue is the only way to correct the problem.

When to Call the Doctor

Doctors recommend you try the "table top test." Try placing the palm of your hand completely flat on a hard surface. If you aren't able to do this, the fingers have contracted to the point where surgery is advised to correct the deformity. The surgery is usually

Viking Disease

Dupuytren's disease is sometimes called Viking disease because it primarily affects people of northern European descent.

successful and the hand can return to normal. However, the disease has been known to recur.

Prevention

Because this condition is heredity, there is no way to prevent it.

FINGERTIP INJURY/AMPUTATION

What It Is

? If you're slicing something with a knife and you aren't careful, you can slice off part of your fingertip. It's a very common injury. The cut may involve only the pad of the finger or may extend through the nail and even into the bone.

Signs and Symptoms

The cut usually will be in the nondominant hand, the one positioning the food or whatever you are cutting with the knife, held in the dominant hand. For example, if you are cutting a tomato with the knife in your right hand (dominant), then the injury would occur to the left fingertip (non-dominant). The fingertip may be cut completely off or still be partially attached. Frequently, there will be considerable bleeding. Wrap your finger in cloth bandages to stop the flow of blood while you seek emergency treatment, but don't wrap it so tightly that you cut off all circulation.

When to Call the Doctor

Any deep cut should be seen immediately by a physician.

How to Treat It

If no bone is exposed, the doctor will anesthetize the finger at its base with a syringe, remove the damaged tissue, clean the wound, and then apply sterile dressings. The finger is placed in a splint to keep it protected and comfortable while it heals. The doctor will probably prescribe antibiotics as well. If the bone is exposed, you'll likely need X-rays, and the doctor will decide whether to shorten the bone slightly to allow room for closing the remaining soft-tissue with stitches. If the nail bed has been cut too, it will need additional stitching to repair. The doctor will also update your tetanus shot, if necessary.

You'll be taught how to change the dressings at home and also how to perform range-of-motion exercises (usually within 48 hours of treatment) to improve circulation and restore movement.

Prevention

Exercise caution when using knives or other cutting tools. Point knife blades down and away from you rather than toward your fingers, use a nonslip cutting surface on which to position the food or material you are cutting, and curl your fingertips down on the object you are cutting. Note that a sharp knife is safer than a dull one because you won't struggle as hard to use it.

Crush Injuries to the Finger

Another common fingertip injury is a crushed finger. This can result in lacerations (torn, ragged wounds), a damaged nail, and even a fracture of the bone in the fingertip. With any crushing injury, you'll typically have pain, bruising, and swelling. If the doctor suspects the bone has been injured, your finger will be X-rayed. A common problem with this type of injury is that blood clots form under the fingernail, causing pressure. The doctor can relieve this by making a small hole in the nail for drainage. The nail bed may also need repair.

FINGERTIP/NAIL INFECTIONS

What It Is

Infections in the fingertip are usually found either in the pad of the tip (where your fingerprint is) or in the area around the edge of the nail. An infection in the pad is called a felon and around the nail is called paronychia. Felons are most common in the index finger or thumb and typically are the result of a puncture wound. These types of wounds are more likely to become infected than cuts because they carry bacteria deeper into the tissue and there is little or no bleeding to clean out the wound.

Paronychia infections can occur after a manicure or from a hangnail or ingrown nail.

Signs and Symptoms

Felons cause severe pain, redness, and swelling in the fingertip pad, and the puncture wound is usually visible. If the pain extends past the tip and into the nearest finger joint, that could indicate a more serious condition such as an infected tendon.

Paronychia causes swelling of the tissues surrounding the fingernail, usually along one side and

Been Fishing?

If you have a fingertip puncture wound from a fishhook, don't try to pull the hook out yourself, as you can cause more damage due to the barb on the end of the hook. Leave the hook in your finger and seek medical attention immediately to have it removed.

the base but sometimes completely around the nail. This condition is painful, too, but not as severe as a felon.

When to Call the Doctor

Call your doctor if you have the symptoms described, because these conditions need prompt medical treatment. Otherwise, there is a risk that the infection could spread to the finger joints and cause serious damage to the bone.

How to Treat It

 In the earliest stages, a fingertip can be treated with antibiotics. But many times

Artificial Nails

The popularity of acrylic nails (artificial nails formed over natural nails to extend them) has led to a few cases of serious nail infections and skin allergies. Sometimes the culprit is methylmethacrylate (MMA), an adhesive the FDA issued a warning about in 1974 but which is still used by some discount salons because it is cheaper than safer acrylics. Many states have outlawed MMA but enforcement is spotty. Avoid salons offering acrylic nails for prices well below the going rate, as this could be an indication that safer adhesive materials are not being used.

a felon must also be drained under local anesthesia to remove the fluid buildup.

Early-stage paronychia is more commonly treated with antibiotics taken for several days. Soaking the finger in warm water for 10 minutes four times a day is also recommended. In later stages, paronychia infections may need to be drained and in severe cases, the nail may have to be removed. The nail should grow out again in several months.

Prevention

Other than exercising care when using sharp objects, it's difficult to prevent puncture wounds and the resulting infections. Proper nail care can help prevent paronychia infections. Avoid nail biting or trimming nails extremely close to the skin. If you have professional manicures, make sure the salon you go to maintains the following standards.

1. Maintains clean, sanitary conditions

2. Is licensed and displays the licenses—with photo ID—of each operator

3. Uses cleaned or single-use implements for each customer

4. Uses small brushes to prevent nail products from coming in contact with skin

FRACTURES OF THE FINGERS, HAND, OR THUMB

What It Is

? Fractures of the fingers, thumb, or hand bones are common. Often your first instinct when you fall is to put out your hands to break your fall. It's common for fingers to be slammed in a door or jammed by a ball during sports. Power saws, drills, and other tools cut fingers just as well as they cut wood or concrete. When you think about all the delicate operations your hands perform in the course of a day, you can see why a broken bone, even a small one in a finger, can be a serious disability if it prevents your hand from working normally.

Signs and Symptoms

Typically, there is swelling, pain, bruising and tenderness at the site of the break. You won't be able to move the finger or thumb completely and it may look unusual—crooked, shorter than normal, or angled in the wrong direction, for example. If the break is to a metacarpal bone (bones in the palm of the hand rather than the finger bones, called phalanges)

Ever Feel Like Punching the Wall?

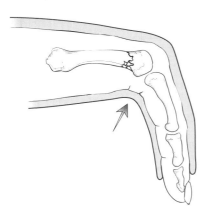 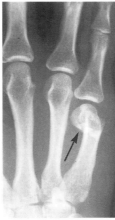

You may not be a boxer, but if you slam your fist into something hard and you break the metacarpal bone leading to the little finger, you've got what's called a boxer's fracture (arrows). Fractures of this bone account for about one third of all hand fractures.

the knuckle may be depressed or one finger may cross over its neighbor when you try to make a partial fist.

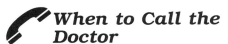

When to Call the Doctor

Call if you have any of the symptoms listed above because a broken bone left untreated can lead to arthritis or other complications. In other parts of the body, it's easier to distinguish a soft-tissue injury, such as a sprain, from a fracture. With fingers, the thumb, or the wrist, the best way for the doctor to know is with an X-ray.

How to Treat It

Treatment depends greatly on the type and severity of the fracture. Most fractures are "nondisplaced," which means the bone is cracked or broken but the pieces are generally in good position for healing. These can be treated with a splint or "buddy taping" the broken finger to an adjoining one. You'll probably have to keep the finger splinted or taped for 3 to 4 weeks.

If the fracture is "displaced," which means the pieces of bone are out of position, or if the fracture is "open," which means the skin is broken over the fractured bone, surgery might be needed to insert pins, plates, screws, or wire to hold the bones in place while the bones heal. Open fractures

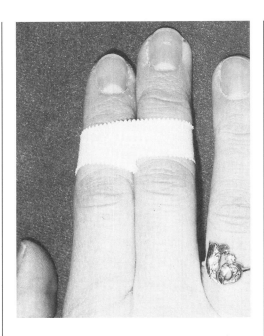

need cleaning during surgery to minimize the risk of bone infection, which can result in permanent problems.

After the splint comes off, you'll need to perform exercises to reduce stiffness and restore maximum mobility, possibly under the direction of an occupational or physical therapist.

Prevention

Take good care of your hands. Don't drink alcohol before using a power saw. Don't disconnect the safety devices on your tools. Resist the urge to punch the wall or window to express your feelings. Be careful of catching gloves, rings, or long sleeves in fast moving tools.

HAND ARTHRITIS

What It Is

? Although arthritis can attack any of the body's joints, appearance-wise it's most noticeable in the hands. While there are many kinds of arthritis, two types primarily affect the hand.

Osteoarthritis (OA) is sometimes called "wear-and-tear" arthritis because the condition involves the wearing away of cartilage, which is the cushioning material attached to the ends of bones, and reduces friction. Occasionally the wear may have resulted from a previous injury such as a fracture that didn't heal properly. OA most often occurs at the base of the thumb, at the middle joint of the finger, or at the joint of the fingertip.

Rheumatoid arthritis (RA) is a disease in which the lining of the joints (synovium) produces chemicals that attack and destroy the joint surfaces. It is most commonly found in the wrist and the finger knuckles. Typically, RA is first diagnosed in middle age, and it affects women two to three times more often than men. Although RA isn't inherited, scientists think some people have certain genes that make them more susceptible, and that the genes are activated by a trigger such as a viral infec-

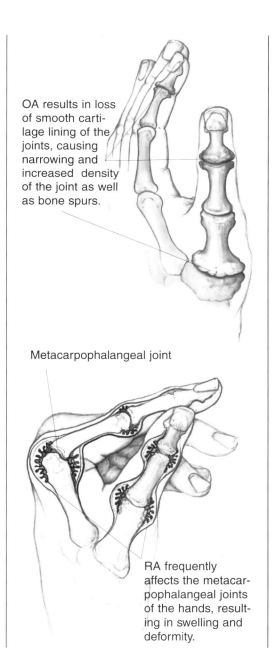

OA results in loss of smooth cartilage lining of the joints, causing narrowing and increased density of the joint as well as bone spurs.

Metacarpophalangeal joint

RA frequently affects the metacarpophalangeal joints of the hands, resulting in swelling and deformity.

tion or some type of environmental factor. The fact that women are more commonly affected than men suggests hormones also play a role.

Signs and Symptoms

Some of the symptoms of the various types of arthritis are similar—stiffness, swelling, pain and loss of motion. With OA, bony growths called nodules sometimes develop in the joints. With RA, as the joints become enlarged or the tendons become irritated, the fingers can be constantly bent, causing the whole hand to take on a deformed appearance. (see figure below.)

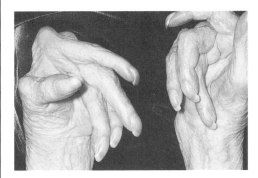

One other distinguishing characteristic of RA is that it usually affects both hands, unlike OA which typically affects just one. Other symptoms of RA are a creaking sound during movement and a soft, lumpy mass on the back of the hand.

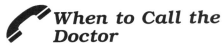

When to Call the Doctor

It's best to consult your doctor when you have these symptoms to rule out other conditions with similar signs and determine which type of arthritis you have. Diagnostic tests may include X-rays, which can show loss of joint space or the presence of nodules, plus blood tests, which can help in identifying RA.

How to Treat It

Treatment to relieve pain and restore function depends on the type of arthritis you have. In general, resting the hand and taking over-the-counter anti-inflammatory medications such as ibuprofen can help reduce swelling and pain. Finger or wrist splints immobilize joints so they can heal. Applying ice packs for 5 to 15 minutes several times a day can help affected joints. Ice, however, should not be applied directly to the skin.

If more pain relief is necessary, your doctor may prescribe stronger medications or steroid injections in the affected parts of the hand. With RA, the doctor may also prescribe medications that slow the progression of the disease. You may be referred to a physical or occupational therapist who can help you change the way you do things with your hands to avoid aggravating the affected joints. For example, using adaptive devices, such as kitchen utensils designed with easy to grip handles, can relieve pressure on arthritic joints.

When other methods fail, doctors sometimes recommend surgery to relieve symptoms and correct deformities. Some of the types of arthritis surgery include draining cysts or removing nodules, replac-ing the damaged joint, or fusing the bones so the joint no longer moves.

Prevention

Currently, there is no cure for RA or OA, although research is ongoing to find cures as well as more effective treatments. If you suffer from a hand injury, seeking treatment promptly and following your doctor's advice may help you avoid post-traumatic arthritis later.

TENDON INJURIES

What It Is

Although it's often called baseball finger, this injury occurs in athletes playing many sports involving balls, including volleyball, basketball, softball, and football. Also called mallet finger, it happens when an object hits the tip of the finger and bends it down farther than it's intended to go. The force of the ball tears the tendon that controls the finger's movement. It can even break off tiny pieces of bone. The injury isn't confined just to athletes. It can happen to anyone whose fingertip meets an unyielding object.

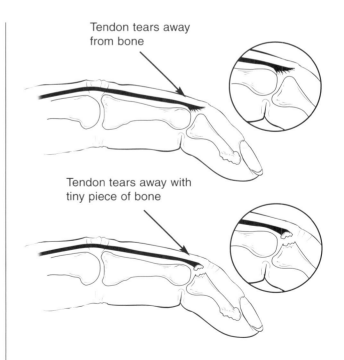

Tendon tears away from bone

Tendon tears away with tiny piece of bone

Signs and Symptoms

This injury can be very painful. Just above the nail, the finger will be red and slightly swollen. You won't be able to straighten your fingertip.

• •

When to Call the Doctor

This condition needs medical treatment; otherwise, the finger can become permanently deformed. It can even cause arthritis in the affected finger later in life.

If you injure your finger, stop playing and immobilize the finger while you apply ice and elevate it above your heart to decrease swelling. Then call your doctor. Treatment is most effective if started within a few days of the injury.

How to Treat It

Your doctor will X-ray the finger and then put it in a straight splint, probably for a minimum of 6 weeks. After that, you'll be able to take the splint off during the day but should wear it at night for another 2 to 4 weeks. When the splint is off, you can start gentle exercises to flex the finger and restore its ability to bend (it will become stiff while in the splint).

While the finger is healing, you should avoid playing sports that could re-injure it. You might be able to participate in limited sports activity after about 6 weeks of treatment with a splint, and return to rigorous sports activity after about 3 months.

In rare cases, if a portion of the bone has broken off, surgical repair may be needed.

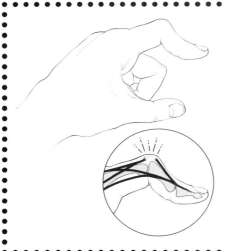

Boutonniere Deformity

This is a rare type of tendon injury in which the middle joint of the finger bends down, but the fingertip end bends up. The word boutonniere is French for "buttonhole," which is what the tendon tear resembles. The treatment is similar to that used for other tendon injuries.

THUMB SPRAIN

What It Is

You're skiing down the slopes when you suddenly lose your balance and your thumb gets in the way. Or maybe you merely tripped over your cat in your living room and put out your hand to break your fall. Either way, the main ligament in your thumb can tear (become sprained). The nickname skier's thumb derives from the fact that skiers are particularly vulnerable. When they fall, they are clutching a ski pole, thus putting extra pressure on the thumb. The ligament may be only partly torn or completely severed.

Signs and Symptoms

Since this ligament serves as a hinge to keep your thumb joint in place, you'll find it difficult to pinch or grasp objects between your thumb and your index finger. Usually, you'll experience pain, but not always. There can also be bruising, tenderness, and swelling.

When to Call the Doctor

If the injury seems minor, you can wait 7 to 10 days and try home treatment first, applying ice two to three times a day for the first 48 hours. If the symptoms persist or are severe, it's wise to see the doctor so the thumb can be splinted until it heals. The doctor can also determine if the ligament is torn partially or completely, since a complete tear may require surgery.

Also Known As. . .

Skier's thumb is sometimes called gamekeeper's thumb. This nickname comes from the sprains that used to occur to England's gamekeepers as a result of their method for killing rabbits!

How to Treat It

In a typical partial tear, you wear a splint for about 4 to 6 weeks. Then you can remove it to do some exercises to restore proper movement but you'll need to put the splint back on when you aren't exercising the thumb. In 2 or 3 more weeks, the swelling and tenderness should be gone and the thumb sprain will be healed. Ice can be applied twice a day in the first 2 or 3 days after the fall to help reduce the swelling.

Prevention

Ski poles with break-away straps can help prevent skier's thumb.

TRIGGER FINGER

What It Is

? No, this isn't a gunslinger's malady. Actually, it's a condition that occurs when a tendon in the finger become irritated. As a result, the tendon swells and catches on its sheath as the finger moves. The tendon may catch and then suddenly release so that you feel a snapping sensation like that of a trigger being released. Also, you may be unable to straighten the finger fully, as if it's about to pull a trigger, so the name has a double meaning. It can happen to any finger but most often affects the middle or the ring fingers.

The precise cause of trigger finger is not known. But people who are at particular risk include those with rheumatoid arthritis, diabetes, or carpal tunnel syndrome.

Signs and Symptoms

The finger hurts when you flex it, and it catches or feels as if it's going out of joint. You may wake up with the finger locked in the palm, although it gradually straightens out during the day. Or you may simply feel swelling and stiffness. Some people also have a painful nodule in the palm near the base of the affected finger.

When to Call the Doctor

Call if the problem interferes with your work or daily activities or if it's painful.

How to Treat It

The doctor may recommend that you rest the finger and take an anti-inflammatory medication such as ibuprofen to relieve the pain. The doctor may also put a splint on the finger to keep it straight. If the symptoms persist, the doctor may recommend a steroid injection, as it can relieve the pain and cure the locking. People with diabetes and rheumatoid arthritis more often need outpatient surgery to correct the problem.

Prevention

In the early stages, if a repetitive motion such as typing aggravates the symptoms, try avoiding these activities.

WRIST FRACTURE

What It Is

? Any of the 10 bones about the wrist (eight carpal bones and the radius and ulna at the end of the forearm), or some combination can be fractured.

The most common wrist fracture is a distal radial fracture, a break at the end of the arm bone (radius) where it joins the wrist. This fracture occurs in people of all ages. Because of the many joints the distal radius makes with the surrounding bones, a variety of fractures can occur, up to 27 different types!

The wrist bone most commonly fractured is the scaphoid bone. If you've fallen on your wrist and you think you've merely sprained it, it's possible that you've actually fractured the scaphoid bone, which is on the thumb side of your wrist. It's easy to be confused because typically when the scaphoid bone breaks, there is little swelling, relatively little pain, and no obvious deformity. It's a common occurrence in sports. If you fall to the ground and the wrist is bent at a 90° angle or greater, the scaphoid bone will likely break. If the angle is less than 90°, the radius is what typically breaks. Wrist fractures also occur as the result of motor vehicle accidents.

Signs and Symptoms

The main symptoms are pain and tenderness to touch—on the thumb side of the wrist if it's a scaphoid fracture or the other side if it's the radius—after a fall or other strong impact. You won't be able to move it as freely as normal, and there may be swelling. Gripping an object may be especially painful.

When to Call the Doctor

If you think you've sprained your wrist, it's a good idea to call your doctor so you can have it X-rayed. X-rays are vital in diagnosing injuries about the wrist. Special X-rays or other special imaging studies may be necessary.

Who's at Risk?

Men between the ages of 20 and 40 are most likely to suffer a fractured wrist from a fall. Children seldom sustain this injury because the growth plate in the wrist takes the force of a fall instead of the wrist bone.

How to Treat It

Most simple fractures heal in a few weeks with splint or cast treatment, but it may take longer if there is a delay in diagnosis and treatment. Sometimes it's difficult to see a wrist fracture on the first set of X-rays. Your doctor will probably immobilize the wrist and thumb with a cast or splint and order further imaging tests in a few weeks. You'll have to have the cast checked regularly to make sure it continues to fit properly and keeps the wrist from moving. After the break heals, physical therapy often is recommended to restore your wrist's strength and range of motion.

If you have a displaced (compound) fracture, which occurs when the break pushes the bone out of alignment, surgery is usually necessary to realign the bone fragments. It's possible that the surgeon will need to use screws, pins, plates, or wires to fix these fractures before the wrist is put into a cast.

Prevention

Wrist guards are recommended for participants in a number of sports to prevent this injury. People who like to roller skate, snowboard, or skate board should consider wearing wrist guards.

WRIST GANGLIONS (CYSTS)

What It Is

If you've noticed a lump on your hand or wrist, don't panic. It's likely a harmless cyst. What causes these fluid-filled sacs to form is not known. Ganglions typically appear on the top of the wrist but sometimes are found on the palm, especially at the base of the fingers. Occasionally, they grow out of the end finger joint. The cysts balloon out between bones and muscles or grow from connective tissues. Sometimes they disappear on their own. People between the ages of 15 and 40 are the most likely to have ganglions.

Who Gets the Bumps?

Wrist ganglions are more common in women than in men. Gymnasts are particularly vulnerable because of the repeated pressure their wrists must withstand.

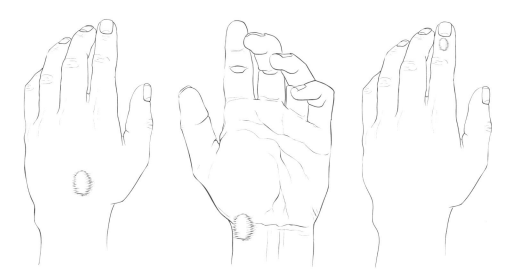

Signs and Symptoms

These cysts can cause pain if they put pressure on nerves and irritate tendons. Smaller ones that sit just under the surface of the skin can be especially painful when you grasp a hard object. Those that grow bigger may not hurt at all, but usually they're unsightly.

If you engage in activities requiring you to move your wrist frequently, the lump will often get bigger. If you give the wrist a chance to rest, however, the lump usually will get smaller.

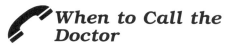

When to Call the Doctor

If the ganglion interferes with your daily activities or causes discomfort, call the doctor.

How to Treat It

The doctor may recommend that you simply rest your wrist and wait to see if the condition improves by itself. A wrist brace or splint can help relieve the symptoms and allow the ganglion to shrink, but this may not make it go away entirely.

Aspiration, which is removal of the fluid with a needle, is a common treatment for bothersome ganglions. The doctor will numb your wrist and insert a needle to draw out the fluid. However, the outer shell of the ganglion remains and, frequently, the cyst reappears. You can have outpatient surgery to remove the ganglion, but even that is no guarantee that it won't come back. Wrist ganglions that have been surgically removed return in 5% to 10% of patients.

HIP AND THIGH

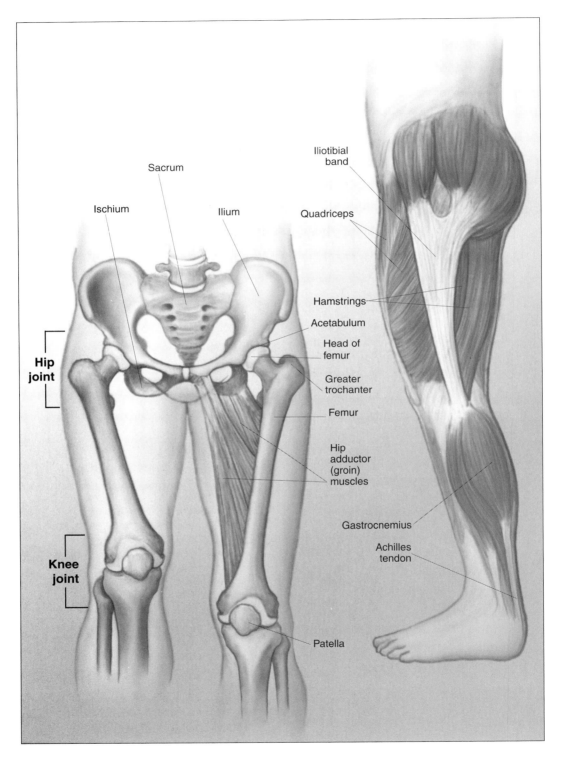

HIP AND THIGH

IF YOU THINK ABOUT SOME OF the contortions of gymnasts or acrobats, you get some idea of just how much movement the hip joint is capable of. You may not be flexible enough to do the splits or curl your legs backwards over your head, but the capacity is there!

The hip is a ball-and-socket joint formed where the rounded end of the thighbone or femur fits into a cup-shaped area, called the acetabulum, in the pelvis. This joint not only allows great range of movement, but it is very strong and is able to bear up under the body's weight and the pounding of a lifetime of walking and running.

Encasing the hip are ligaments that surround the joint and hold it together. Over the ligaments are tendons that attach muscles in the buttocks, thighs, and pelvis to the bones. These muscles control hip movement. Fluid-filled pockets called bursal sacs are located in strategic spots around the hip to provide cushioning and reduce friction in the moving parts.

The hip joint is lined with a thin layer of cartilage, a rubbery substance that provides cushioning between bones so they won't rub together. The cartilage can wear away as people age. This condition is called osteoarthritis (OA) and is one of the most common ailments of the hip. Most people over 55 have some degree of osteoarthritis visible on X-rays, but only a small portion have pain as a result.

As with other parts of the musculoskeletal system, exercise can go a long way toward keeping the hip sturdy and flexible. Because it is a strong joint and well protected, the hip isn't as prone to injury as are more fragile parts of the body.

DEVELOPMENTAL DISLOCATION (DYSPLASIA) OF THE HIP

What It Is

? A baby born with a hip in which the ball on top of thighbone (femur) is not held firmly in the socket is said to have developmental dysplasia (dislocation) of the hip (DDH). The head of the femur may be loose in the socket, or it may be completely dislocated. The looseness may worsen as the child grows. When the condition is detected at birth, it usually can be corrected with nearly normal results. But if detection is delayed until the child begins walking, the treatment becomes more complicated and the prospect of making the hip normal is not as good.

Signs and Symptoms

Pediatricians routinely check newborns for DDH during the first examination and at subsequent well-baby check-ups. Early detection is important because the condition is much easier to treat if it's caught before a child starts to walk. DDH is three times as likely to occur in the left hip. Sometimes children who are born with

Who is Most Affected?

DDH can run in families. It's also more likely to affect girls and first-born children, and it is more common in Caucasians of northern European ancestry and Native Americans. It is rarely seen in African-American children.

torticollis, a condition in which the head is tilted also have DDH. (See p 269 for more information.)

Infants born in the breech position, especially with their feet up by their shoulders, are at risk for DDH. The American Academy of Pediatrics recommends that newborn girls who are breech or who have other risk factors should undergo an ultrasound or other imaging of their hips to look for the condition.

When to Call the Doctor

If your baby receives regular check-ups, in most cases your doctor should find the problem before you notice symptoms. And only rarely does a hip found to be normal at birth become abnormal later. But you should certainly call the doctor if you notice that your baby's legs are of different lengths, the thigh skin folds are uneven, or the baby has less mobility or flexibility on one side. In children who have begun to walk, limping, toe walking, and a waddling or "duck-like" gait can all be signs of DDH.

How to Treat It

Treatment depends on the age of the baby when DDH is detected. If it's found in the first 6 months of age, the baby is placed in a soft position-ing device, a Pavlik harness (see figure), to keep the femur in the socket until the socket forms. If that doesn't work in 2 to 3 weeks, the doctor may have to anes-thetize the child and examine and manipulate the hip into proper position, then put the child into a body cast.

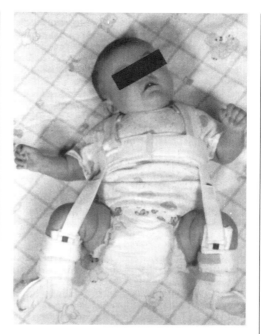

If the child is older than 6 to 9 months, a special cast, called a spica cast, is used. A child left untreated until after age 2 will need surgery to correct what by that time is likely to be a serious condition that may affect the hip into adulthood.

GROIN STRAIN

What It Is

Your groin muscles, techni-cally called the hip adductor muscles, are on the inside of your thighs and provide the ability and strength to bring your legs together. If these muscles are strained, it can be quite painful.

Signs and Symptoms

You'll feel a sudden, sharp pain and have difficulty or be unable to draw your leg inward. In a few days, there also may be bruising and swelling, depending on how severely the muscle is stretched or torn. If the muscle is torn (ruptured), you won't be able to draw your leg up toward your chest at all.

How to Treat It

1. Simple strains can be treated at home with the RICE (Rest, Ice, Compression, Elevation) method.

2. Keep off of your leg as much as possible for the first day or two.

3. Apply an ice pack for 20 minutes, two to three times a day.

4. Press on the muscle when applying the ice to provide some compression, as this helps reduce swelling. Wrap an elastic bandage around your groin area when you aren't icing it.

5. Raise your thigh above the level of your heart, whenever possible. Try lying down with your leg propped up on pillows or on your side with the injured side up.

6. Take an anti-inflammatory medication such as ibuprofen to reduce the pain and inflammation.

When to Call the Doctor

If the pain is severe and you can't draw your leg up, call your doctor. You may have torn the mus-

A Word About Stress Fractures

Groin pain may also be a sign of a stress fracture of the hip. This is often the result of an overuse injury such as running on a hard surface. The fracture can be in the neck of the femur where it hooks into the hip joint, or more rarely, in the pelvic bone. The ache may be felt in the hip but it can also be in the groin.

To treat stress fractures in the hip, doctors recommend you curtail any strenuous activity such as running or jogging. Once the diagnosis is made, your doctor may put you on crutches for a few weeks until the fracture is well on its way to healing.

cle, not just strained it. Your doctor may have you use crutches until the pain or limp decreases, usually about 6 to 8 weeks, and may recommend physical therapy. Pain that is not severe but lasts longer than 3 days also warrants a call to the doctor. Other conditions can cause pain in this area and could be the reason the symptoms are continuing.

Prevention

It's important to perform warm-up and cool-down exercises before and after vigorous activity. Conditioning exercises that make the thigh muscles (quadriceps) stronger and more flexible will also make them less likely to suffer strains. Build up gradually when you start training for a new activity such as distance running.

HIP ARTHRITIS

What It Is

? Arthritis, an inflammation of the joint, is the most frequent cause of chronic hip pain.

Here are the three most common forms of arthritis:

1. Osteoarthritis (OA) usually affects people over age 50. After many years of movement, the cartilage that cushions the hip bones literally wears away, allowing the bones to rub against each other, causing inflammation and pain.

2. Rheumatoid arthritis (RA) is a disease in which the synovial membrane, a thin, smooth tissue that lines and lubricates the hip joint, becomes inflamed. As a result, too much fluid is produced causing damage to the cartilage. RA typically affects multiple joints, not just the hip.

3. Post-traumatic arthritis sometimes follows an injury to the hip such as a fracture or dislocation. Again, damage to the cartilage causes friction and pain.

Signs and Symptoms

Typically, you feel a dull, aching pain in the groin, the buttocks, or the outer side of the thigh. You may have pain and stiffness when you get up in the morning that improves with moderate activity. The pain and stiffness worsen if you try more vigorous activity, however. A limp is common, and you won't be able to move your hip as far as normal.

When to Call the Doctor

Stiffness and pain in the hip could be a sign of arthritis but could also be caused by an infection or other serious problem. If you have these symptoms for more than a few days or if the pain is severe, consult your doctor.

How to Treat It

You and your doctor can discuss an array of treatments—both medical and physical—that will work best for your particular type of arthritis. Treatment can include medications for pain relief, physical therapy, and use of a cane when walking to ease the pressure of weight bearing.

When other measures offer no relief from pain after about 3 months of nonsurgical treatment, your doctor may recommend hip replacement surgery, which can eliminate pain and increase your range of motion. (See below for more information on this surgery.)

Prevention

If you are at risk for OA, it's best to avoid pounding activities, such as running on cement or asphalt. Doctors don't yet know how to prevent RA.

HIP REPLACEMENT SURGERY

The first hip replacement surgery was performed in 1960 and is considered one of the major medical breakthroughs of our time. Advancements in materials, surgical techniques, and prosthesis design have steadily improved the success rate. More than 160,000 total hip replacements are performed each year, and in only 10% of those cases, does the hip have to be replaced a second time.

What It Is

Hip replacement surgery or total hip arthroplasty (THA) is reserved for people for whom simpler measures haven't worked. Nonsurgical treatments for relieving the pain and stiffness of arthritis include use of canes or walkers, anti-inflammatory medications, and physical therapy. If, after trying these or other remedies, you are unable to maintain daily activities such as walking or sitting in a chair because of persistent pain, hip replacement surgery may be the solution. The goal of THA is to relieve pain and improve mobility.

It used to be that THA was recommended primarily for people over 60. The problem with offering THA to younger patients was that an artificial hip (prosthesis) didn't hold up as well under the more active lifestyle of younger adults. But new technology has produced better prostheses that can withstand more stress. The main drawback is that after 15 or 20 years, the prosthesis wears out and must be replaced. Despite this drawback, THA can so improve a patient's lifestyle, that doctors are recommending it more frequently to their younger patients so they can enjoy the benefits of the surgery during the more active period of their lives. And, if they avoid high-impact activities, patients can extend the life of the prosthesis.

How Hip Replacement Surgery Is Done

Hip replacement is a major surgery and is done in a hospital, usually with general anesthesia, although spinal anesthesia, which numbs you from the waist down, is sometimes used. In a THA, a surgeon removes the damaged hip joint and replaces it with a prosthesis. The procedure takes a few hours.

Although hip prostheses come in a variety of designs and materials, they all have two basic parts that mimic your own hip. There is a ball made of a highly polished strong metal and a socket or cup made with a durable plastic. The socket may have an outer metal shell. Usually, a type of special cement is used to secure the prosthesis to the part of your natural bone that remains. In younger, more active patients, surgeons sometimes use a non-cemented prosthesis that is coat-

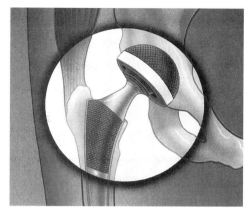

ed with a textured or bone-like substance that allows the bone to grow into the prosthesis. Sometimes a combination of a cemented ball and a non-cemented socket is used. Your surgeon will discuss with you which type of prosthesis is best for you.

What to Expect After Surgery

Most people who undergo THA find their pain dramatically reduced or eliminated. They also enjoy major improvements in mobility, although certain activities must be permanently avoided such as high-impact sports and jogging. For people who are overweight, the surgeon may recommend shedding some pounds because excess weight may cause the prosthesis to wear out sooner or to loosen and become painful.

After surgery, you usually remain in the hospital for 3 to 5 days and will probably begin walking with a walker or crutches beginning the day after surgery. After the hospital stay, you typically will be transferred to a skilled nursing facility for 1 to 2 weeks. During that time, a physical therapist teaches you hip strengthening exercises to perform at home.

Recovery continues at home for several weeks. Initially, you'll need help with chores such as cooking, bathing, shopping, and laundry. If you live alone, the hospital or our doctor can help you make arrangements in advance for some help at home. Usually you can resume light activity, including walking and performing household tasks, within 3 to 6 weeks. Precautions should be taken to avoid falls and injuries to the new hip during the recovery period. (See p 38 for tips on avoiding falls.)

Passing the Metal Detector

Artificial hips can set off metal detectors used for security in airports and other places. Your surgeon can give you a Medic-Alert card, confirming that you have an artificial hip, should you ever need one to show security guards.

Maintaining an active lifestyle with regular exercise will keep your hip strong and flexible. But you should avoid activities such as jogging or skiing that put repeated stress on the hip. Opt instead for such activities as swimming, biking, golf, or doubles tennis.

HIP BURSITIS

What It Is

? The hip is one of several joints in the body that can suffer from bursitis. A bursa is a small fluid-filled sac that provides a cushion between bones, tendons, and muscles. Several bursae can be found around the outer area of the hip near the place where the thighbone (femur) joins the pelvis (see figure). A common cause of hip pain is an inflammation in one of the bursa.

Who Gets Bursitis?

Hip bursitis can affect you at any age, but it is more common in women and middle-aged or elderly people.

When the bursitis is in the hip, it is referred to as trochanteric bursitis because the hip end of the femur is called the trochanter.

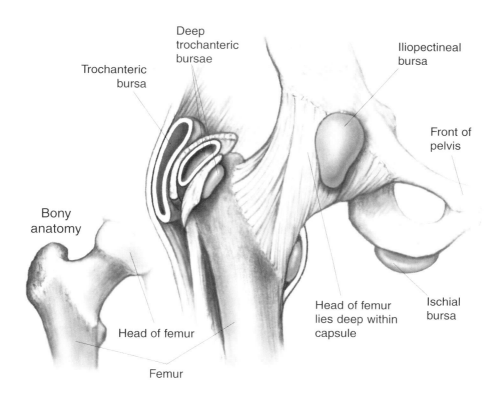

Trochanteric bursa

Deep trochanteric bursae

Iliopectineal bursa

Front of pelvis

Bony anatomy

Head of femur

Head of femur lies deep within capsule

Ischial bursa

Head of femur

Femur

Hip bursitis has many possible causes:

1. Repetitive stress or overuse injuries

2. Lying on one side of the body for an extended period (perhaps while recovering from a different injury)

3. Excessive or prolonged pressure on the hip such as from standing for lengthy periods

4. Uneven leg lengths

5. Spine disease such as scoliosis

6. Rheumatoid arthritis (RA)

7. Previous hip surgery, especially if prosthetic devices were implanted

Signs and Symptoms

The main symptom is aching pain, which is usually focused on the outside of the upper thigh, just over the point of the hip. The pain may radiate down the outside of the thigh as far as the knee. The pain is worse when you lie down or roll over on the affected side. It may be difficult for you to sleep, walk, climb stairs, or sit or stand too long. The pain also is worse when you first stand up after sitting or lying down. Then you may feel better after a few steps. But the discomfort typically recurs if you walk for half an hour or more.

When to Call the Doctor

Call if the pain is severe or lasts for more than 2 or 3 days. Based on your symptoms and the location of the pain, your doctor is generally able to make the diagnosis but additional tests may be ordered if he or she suspects you have underlying conditions or injuries causing the hip pain. For example, bone spurs or calcium deposits can contribute to bursitis. Particularly if the pain persists after initial treatment, the doctor may want X-rays or a magnetic resonance imaging (MRI) test to detect these or other conditions.

How to Treat It

If the cause is overuse, the primary treatment is to rest so the hip has time to heal. This doesn't mean taking to your bed, but rather to modify your daily activities and exercise routine so you don't exert as much stress on the hip. Depending on the severity of your symptoms, your doctor may also recommend using a cane to reduce the pressure on the hip. The length of time you'll need to use the cane depends on your symptoms.

An anti-inflammatory medication such as ibuprofen not only relieves the pain but helps reduce the inflammation. You can also apply an ice pack over the point of your hip for 15 to 20 minutes, two or three times a day. Your doctor may also recommend physical therapy.

If the pain persists after you've tried these steps, your doctor may recommend a corticosteroid injection. This treatment usually relieves the symptoms. Surgery for hip bursitis is rare.

If the bursitis occurs because your legs are of different lengths, you can be fitted for a lift in your shoe so you don't lean to one side when you walk.

Prevention

Try to avoid prolonged standing or repetitive tasks that put stress on your hip muscles. Also, do exercises designed to strengthen and stretch the muscles in your hip and lower back. If you are overweight, losing some pounds will also help reduce the pressure on your hip.

HIP DISLOCATION

What It Is

A hip dislocation—when the thighbone (femur) pops out of the hip socket—is a serious medical emergency. The bone itself isn't damaged as in a fracture, but the separation of the femur from its socket causes damage to the surrounding tissues. Often the cause of the injury is a motor vehicle crash. Sometimes a fall from a ladder or other high place is the cause.

Signs and Symptoms

Severe pain and the inability to move the leg are classic signs. In addition, the person may report loss of feeling in the foot or ankle; this is due to nerve damage. Other injuries are common as well.

In 90% of dislocations, the head of the femur is pushed out and back, causing the hip and leg to twist toward the middle of the body. In the other 10%, the leg will twist out and away from the body because the femur was thrust out of the socket in a forward direction.

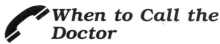

When to Call the Doctor

Call 9-1-1 immediately! Don't try to move the injured person, but keep him or her warm with blankets until help arrives.

How to Treat It

If the dislocation is not accompanied by complications such as fractured bones, the patient can be anesthetized so the surgeon can manipulate the bones back into their proper position. If there are complications, surgery will be necessary to set the bones and reposition the hip.

Sometimes traction, from the hip to the heel, is necessary for a short time following a hip dislocation. Traction may be followed by controlled exercises on a special machine (a physical therapy modality called continuous passive motion) that moves the patient's leg. Then the patient progresses to crutches and finally to a cane until the limp disappears.

A hip dislocation can have long-term consequences because it damages the nerves and muscles around the hip joint. The most serious consequences occur if the blood supply to the head of the femur is interrupted and, as a result, it dies. For this reason, arthritis can develop in people who have suffered this injury.

Prevention

Wearing a seatbelt greatly minimizes your chances of dislocating your hip. Also, learn to prevent falls. (See "Preventing Falls" on p 38 for a checklist of tips.)

HIP FRACTURE

What It Is

Hip fractures are primarily a problem for elderly people, with women affected two to three times more often than men. Ninety percent of hip fractures are caused by a fall. The rest are typically from injuries sustained in motor vehicle crashes, industrial accidents, or other incidents involving severe trauma. About half the time, people who are diagnosed with a hip fracture due to a fall actually fell because the hip fractured first.

Age is the biggest risk factor because bones thin and weaken as you get older. As the population in the United States ages, the incidence of hip fractures will grow. After age 50, the risk doubles each decade. But it's really people 65 and older who are most affected; 90% of all hip fractures occur in this age group.

Heredity is a factor, too. If your family has a history of broken bones in later life, you are at greater risk. Also, Caucasian women are two to three times more likely to break a hip than Hispanic or African-American women. Being small boned or being very slender also makes you

Who Recovers?

- *About 25% recover completely; the rest may have a permanent limp, persistent pain, altered balance, and difficulty climbing stairs.*

- *About 30% to 40% cannot live independently.*

- *About 20% of elderly patients die within a year of the injury because pre-existing problems with their heart, lungs, or kidneys can become worse.*

more vulnerable. People who smoke or use alcohol excessively increase their risk, too.

Besides the fact that bones weaken with age, elderly people are prone to falls if they are taking certain types of medication, suffer from dizziness, dementia, or strokes.

Signs and Symptoms

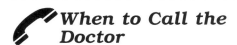

If you fall and then can't walk because you unable to bear weight, you should suspect a hip fracture. The leg may also appear shortened or twisted. A few people report pain, mostly in the knee.

When to Call the Doctor

If you strongly suspect someone has suffered a hip fracture, don't move him or her. Call 9-1-1 immediately. Keep the person warm with blankets until help arrives.

Falls are not uncommon among the elderly, and at least some pain and stiffness as a result are natural and aren't necessarily signs of a broken bone. If the person isn't able to put weight on the affected leg or feels pain when moving the leg, see a doctor for an X-ray to determine if there is a fracture.

Who's at Risk?

Nearly half of the women who reach age 90 have suffered from a hip fracture. The odds of avoiding it are better for short women because the risk of hip fracture in those who are 5' 8" and taller is twice that of women under 5' 2". Doctors speculate the reason is that taller women fall from a greater height, causing the hip to sustain a more severe blow.

How to Treat It

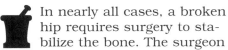

In nearly all cases, a broken hip requires surgery to stabilize the bone. The surgeon inserts pins or other devices to hold it in place until it heals. If this is done within the first 24 to 48 hours, the complications that come from bed rest can be reduced.

The length of stay in the hospital and the recovery period afterward varies, depending on the severity of the fracture, age of the patient, and overall health. All patients require canes or walkers for several months after the surgery, and nearly half will need to use them permanently.

Prevention

✔ Everything from climbing the stairs to getting out of the bathtub can be a fall waiting to happen. But there are lots of measures you can take to reduce your risk such as eliminating hazards in your home, wearing the right shoes, exercising to maintain agility and balance, and using over-the-counter drugs cautiously. (See "Preventing Falls" on p 38 for a checklist of tips.)

Also, you'll be less likely to suffer a fracture in a fall if your bones are strong. Eating a diet with adequate calcium and getting the right kinds of exercise can help you significantly lower your risk. (See p 19 for the "Healthy Bones Diet.")

HIP PAIN IN ADOLESCENTS

What It Is

? In adolescents, growth spurts can cause susceptibility to changes in the skeletal structure. That's why children's bones have growth plates or areas at the ends of bones that grow but respond to forces placed on them. In children with a condition called slipped capital femoral epiphysis (SCFE), the head of the thighbone (femur) slips off of the main part of the bone at the growth plate. It looks a bit like ice cream falling off an ice cream cone.

The slipping occurs after a series of microstresses that allow the ball of the hip to gradually slip out of place in relation to the thighbone. Boys are at greater risk than girls, as are young athletes. Obesity is a risk factor, too.

Most kids who have SCFE are heavier than the average in their age group. There also is a greater incidence among African-Americans.

A small percentage of adolescents with SCFE have a hormonal disorder that affects the strength of the growth plate.

Signs and Symptoms

Pain that gets worse with physical activity is the main symptom, along with a limp. The pain is typically in the groin area, but some patients complain of pain farther down the thigh and into the knee. The pain can develop gradually or may occur suddenly, preventing the ability to bear any weight.

The average age for girls to be diagnosed with SCFE is 12, with the typical age range being 10 to 14 years. With boys, the typical age range is 11 to 16 years with the average age being 13. Between 20% and 30% of adolescents with SCFE eventually have it in both hips.

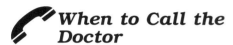

When to Call the Doctor

Call the doctor if your adolescent complains of hip or leg pain or is limping and unable to walk for more than 2 days.

How to Treat It

Youngsters diagnosed with SCFE need surgery to stabilize the bone to prevent further slippage until the growth plate closes. The surgeon usually places a pin in the joint while the child is under general anesthesia. The child will be instructed in how to use crutches, allowing only the toes to touch the ground while the hip heals, usually in about 6 weeks.

Prevention

The only prevention measure doctors can recommend is avoiding obesity.

LEGG-CALVÉ-PERTHES DISEASE

What It Is

Legg-Calvé-Perthes disease (LCPD) is a hip condition affecting the top of the thighbone (femoral head) where it connects to the hip socket. What happens in this condition is that, for reasons doctors aren't yet sure about, the bone in the femoral head dies due to an interruption of the blood supply. The bone then becomes brittle and may collapse like a dimple on a ping-pong ball, eventually causing wear-and-tear arthritis (osteoarthritis) in the hip at a young age. Better long-term results from treatment are possible when the child is under age 6 at diagnosis.

Doctors do not know the cause of this condition. However, since it is common in very active boys, trauma (such as falls or jumping) may be a factor. LCPD most often appears in children between ages 4 and 8, but it can occur in children as young as 2 or as old as 12. In 90% of the cases, only one hip is affected, and when both hips are involved, it happens at different times. It's four times more likely to affect boys than girls, and only rarely affects African-American children.

Signs and Symptoms

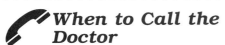 With LCPD, your child typically will report an aching hip or thigh pain. Often, the pain starts first in the knee or thigh and later moves to the groin. The child will also limp from time to time, and the limp will get worse with more activity. Or you may notice that the limp gets worse by the end of the day.

When to Call the Doctor

It's not unusual for children to complain of pain in the hip, knee, or pelvis. The cause can be an injury from sports or other physical activity, or it could be a case of "growing pains." But if your child complains about pain or limps for more than a few days, it's wise to call the doctor. The sooner kids get treatment, the better their chances for a good outcome.

How to Treat It

It's possible for the bone in the head of the femur to begin healing itself after it dies. But doctors can't make that happen, they can only let nature take its course. Children's bones have an amazing ability to repair themselves, certainly more so than adults. The doctor may prescribe physical therapy and a night brace to keep the leg in a certain position as the new growth occurs in order to mold the ball of the femur into its normal spherical shape. This is called containment treatment. Unfortunately, the process can take several months. Periodic X-rays and physical examinations can chart the bone's progress.

In some cases, surgery may be required to change the shape of the socket and deepen it. Occasionally the surgery may be needed to reposition the upper femur. Surgery is more likely to be necessary in children older than 6 years.

Prevention

There is no known prevention for this condition.

What are Growing Pains?

Preschool and school-age children sometimes complain of unexplained aches in their hips or legs, often in the evening or during the night when they are trying to sleep. Some people refer to these as "growing pains," but there is no evidence that growth is the cause. Some research shows a link to intense physical activity. The pain is harmless and eventually disappears as children age. But growing pains can cause real discomfort, but you can ease the pain by stretching and massaging the affected muscles and applying warm compresses.

MUSCLE STRAIN

What It Is

? Whether you are a top athlete or just play an occasional game of pick-up basketball or go water-skiing on the weekend, you may have experienced a strain to your thigh muscles. The hamstrings are the three muscles at the back of the thigh. The quadriceps are the four muscles on the top or front of the thigh. Hamstring injuries are the more common injury of the two, but both occur frequently during sports and can be very debilitating. These injuries can also occur during jobs that require repeated squatting and lifting, gardening, for example.

Most at risk are people who engage in activities or sports that involve running with quick stops and starts. Gymnasts are especially vulnerable to hamstring strains because of the extreme stretching some of their movements require.

Signs and Symptoms

With a hamstring strain, you may feel a "pull" or a "pop" and notice pain at the back of the thigh. If it's a mild strain, you may be able to continue running or playing but the muscle may ache later. If the pain is severe enough that you have to

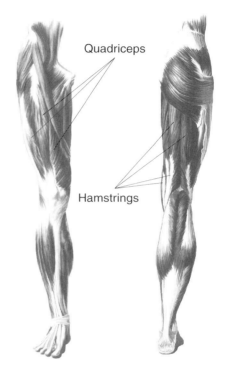

Quadriceps

Hamstrings

stop, that's a sign that you've done more damage. In a few days you're also likely to notice bruising under the skin.

With a quadriceps strain, you may feel a sudden pain on the top of the thigh, although you might not notice it until after you've stopped playing and try to straighten your leg. Or the pain may be so severe that you can't continue playing. Sometimes the quadriceps strain is the result of a direct blow during a contact sport.

In both types of strains, it's important to treat them promptly and for as long as it takes for the muscles to heal; otherwise, the problem is likely to recur.

How to Treat It

With any kind of strain, the muscle either stretches, tears, or ruptures. Treatment methods depend on the severity of the strain. Start the RICE (Rest, Ice, Compression, Elevation) treatment at home as soon as you notice the injury:

1. Keep off of your leg as much as possible for the first day or two.

2. Apply an ice pack for 20 minutes two to three times a day.

3. Press on the muscle when applying the ice to provide some compression, as this helps to reduce swelling. Wrap an elastic bandage around the thigh when you aren't icing it. It's also okay to apply the ice over the top of the bandage.

4. Raise the thigh above the level of your heart, whenever possible. Try lying down with your leg propped up on pillows.

Prompt treatment could shave days or even weeks off your rehabilitation period. Recovery from a simple strain can take 3 to 5

days, but several weeks are required for severe cases. To reduce pain and inflammation during this time, take an anti-inflammatory medication such as ibuprofen.

After the first few days and as the pain decreases, you can begin gentle exercises to strengthen and stretch the injured muscles to keep them flexible. Later, as you resume activities, it may be helpful to wear a support, such as a neoprene sleeve, which has the added benefit of retaining heat.

When to Call the Doctor

If you have pain and are unable to bear weight or walk without difficulty and these symptoms last more than 2 days without improvement, call your doctor. He may have you use crutches, prescribe stronger anti-inflammatory medication, and/or start you on physical therapy.

Prevention

Always perform some warm-up exercises before beginning more rigorous activity and cool-down exercises at the end. This makes the muscles more supple and less vulnerable to strains.

Sciatica (Herniated Disk)

What It Is

? Sciatica is actually a symptom rather a problem itself. It's a distinctive and severe pain that runs from the hip into the thigh via the sciatic nerve, the largest one in your body. This nerve originates in the lower back and branches out through both hips into the legs.

The culprit often is a herniated lumbar disk—a disk in the lower back. It's sometimes called a slipped disk but that's really a misnomer because the disk itself doesn't slip out of place. As we age, cracks may form in the bone and allow some of the disk's soft, inside material to protrude out into the spinal column. This places pressure on the nerve roots that make up the sciatic nerve and causes the pain. Younger people sometimes develop a herniated disk as the result of an injury, for example, a blow to the back during a football game. Less common causes of sciatica include infections and tumors.

Signs and Symptoms

Sciatica is a pain, often severe, that radiates from the lower back down one or both buttocks into the backs of the legs and sometimes into spe-

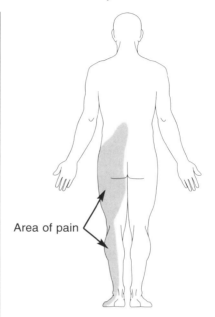

Area of pain

cific areas of the foot and toes. The pain may begin suddenly or it may develop gradually. Sometimes it starts in the lower back but then disappears when it shifts to the legs. Certain activities such as sitting, walking, or even sneezing and coughing can make it worse. You may get some pain relief when you lie down on your back with a pillow under your knees or lie in a fetal position on your side.

How to Treat It

If the pain is not severe, rest for a couple of days and take anti-inflammatory medication such as ibuprofen.

You can also try applying ice packs or heat packs for 20 minutes.

When to Call the Doctor

If the symptoms don't improve in 2 to 3 days or the pain is severe, call your doctor. Most cases of sciatica caused by a herniated disk can be treated without any lasting effects. Depending on the patient, the doctor may prescribe nonsteroidal anti-inflammatory medications, muscle relaxants, narcotic medications or steroids to provide pain relief in the first few days. One to 3 days of bed rest is advisable. After that, you can limit the amount of time you sit, stand or walk, and take frequent rests.

Recently, there has been a lot of interest in complementary and alternative medicine technologies to relieve sciatica. Various herbal and homeopathic compounds have anti-inflammatory effects. Acupuncture has also been effective in relieving pain.

With proper treatment, the great majority of sciatica sufferers get relief from their symptoms within 6 weeks and only 10% still have significant symptoms beyond 3 months. Surgery is seldom necessary.

Prevention

Keep your back healthy with back strengthening exercises and avoid activities that cause back injuries such as lifting heavy loads improperly.

SNAPPING HIP

What It Is

Do you feel a snapping or popping sensation when you walk or rotate your hip? The likely cause is the aptly named "snapping hip"—or its technical name, iliotibial band syndrome. It occurs when the normally painless action of the tendon sliding over the bony prominences at the end of the thighbone (femur)

becomes painful because of swelling in the bursal sac, a fluid-filled pocket that, when working properly, reduces friction. The snapping feeling is not only painful but annoying.

Signs and Symptoms

The snapping sensation may be felt in the groin when the hip extends from a flexed position such as when you rise from a chair. Some people notice it when they are lying with the affected side up and happen to move the leg. If the snapping is the result of cartilage tears, the condition can be more disabling and cause pain. You may feel the need to grab for support when it happens.

The Link to Bursitis

Some people with snapping hip also develop bursitis as the bursa located between the bone and the snapping tendon becomes irritated.

When to Call the Doctor

If the condition isn't particularly bothersome, you may just want reassurance from your doctor that the symptoms you have aren't cause for alarm. Pain, however, definitely merits a visit to the doctor.

How to Treat It

If you have pain, an anti-inflammatory medication such as ibuprofen can help.

You also may be advised to avoid activities that aggravate the problem until the symptoms subside. Stretching exercises can help, too. In extreme cases, the doctor may recommend a corticosteroid injection.

Prevention

Remember the mantra "If it hurts, don't do it." Early signs of discomfort are a signal to avoid a particular activity that is straining the hip.

TRANSIENT SYNOVITIS IN CHILDREN

What It Is

Young children sometimes experience hip pain that is caused by a condition called transient synovitis. It's technically a type of arthritis in that it is an inflammation and swelling of the joint. Fortunately, it usually goes away in a few days with no lasting side effects.

Synovitis is the term used to describe a condition in which the synovial membrane, a thin smooth tissue that lines the hip joint, produces too much fluid.

Doctors don't know the actual cause of the problem, although it may result from a mild injury to the hip at an age when the hip joint hasn't fully developed or it may be a response to a recent viral illness.

Transient synovitis usually affects children ages 2 to 5 years old. It affects boys two to three times more often than girls.

Signs and Symptoms

When the child wakes up, he starts walking with a limp or may even refuse to walk. If he's old enough to communicate with you, he'll likely complain of a pain in the groin area high on the thigh. Sometimes, after the child moves around for a while, the symptoms improve, but they may get worse again by the end of the day.

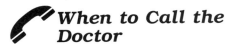

When to Call the Doctor

Any limp or hip pain, especially if it is accompanied by a fever, should be reported to your doctor because it could be due to a variety of causes, some of which need prompt medical treatment.

How to Treat It

A few days of bed rest and an anti-inflammatory medication usually clears up the symptoms, which can last from 3 days to 2 weeks. Your child should be monitored carefully for fever or other illness. If either develop, call the doctor as these could signal a bacterial infection or other more serious condition.

KNEE AND LOWER LEG

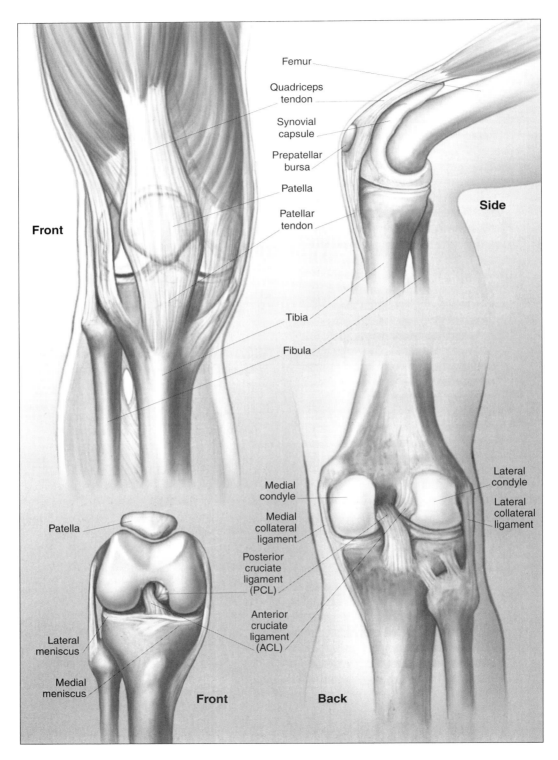

Femur

Quadriceps
tendon

Synovial
capsule

Prepatellar
bursa

Patella

Patellar
tendon

Side

Front

Tibia

Fibula

Lateral
condyle

Lateral
collateral
ligament

Medial
condyle

Medial
collateral
ligament

Posterior
cruciate
ligament
(PCL)

Anterior
cruciate
ligament
(ACL)

Patella

Lateral
meniscus

Medial
meniscus

Front

Back

KNEE AND LOWER LEG

THE KNEE IS THE BODY'S biggest joint. Even so, it's not always able to stand up to the abuse we give it. About 11 million people a year visit a doctor for knee problems and injuries.

The knee has just three bones—the ends of the thighbone (femur) and leg bone (tibia) plus the kneecap (patella), which slides in a groove on the end of the femur and protects the front of the joint. The joint is held together by a network of muscles, ligaments, and tendons. These serve as shock absorbers, helping the knee withstand the strain from walking, running, jumping, dancing, skiing, in-line skating, contact sports, and lifting large objects, among other things.

There are four major ligaments in the knee, two of which are referred to as cruciate because they crisscross each other to form an X inside the knee joint. The one closer to the front (anterior) of the knee is the anterior cruciate ligament (ACL), and the one toward the back is called the pos-

terior cruciate ligament (PCL). Both of these can be injured during sports. The other two major ligaments are the medial collateral ligament (MCL) on the inner side of the knee, and the lateral collateral ligament (LCL) on the outside. Of these two, the medial is more easily injured than the lateral.

Although its bone structure seems simple, the knee can have a multitude of problems. During activity, ligaments and tendons can tear. So can cartilage, the cushioning tissue between the bones. Among the most common problems in the lower leg are shin-splints (muscle pain) and stress fractures. Both are related to overtraining. Injury to the ligaments often is serious because these tough bands of tissue can be partly or completely torn during physical activity, especially in certain sports that involve jumping, pivoting, and sudden stops. Sometimes surgery and lengthy periods of rehabilitation are needed before injured athletes can return to their sports. Knees also are vulnerable to osteoarthritis

Preventing Traumatic Knee Injury

1. *Keep your thigh muscles (hamstrings in back and quadriceps in front) strong and flexible through specific exercises so they'll be better able to support and protect your knee joint.*

2. *Warm up your muscles with stretches before exercising.*

3. *Wear appropriate kneepads when playing sports or engaging in activities such as in-line skating.*

4. *If you are overweight, lose some pounds.*

5. *Avoid sudden increases in the intensity of your workouts.*

6. *Wear shoes that fit properly and provide good support.*

7. *Learn proper techniques for landing from a jump, pivoting, and stopping during sports.*

(commonly called "wear-and-tear") arthritis. Trauma can cause the bones to fracture or dislocate. And that's just the short list of what can go wrong!

Many knee problems can be treated nonsurgically with rest, ice, compression, and elevation—a simple treatment plan often referred to as RICE. Others require surgery. Surgical techniques, using new methods and materials, are constantly improving so that most patients are usually able to return to normal activity and even resume participation in sports. Older people who suffer from osteoarthritis can get relief from chronic pain with complete knee joint replacements.

ANTERIOR CRUCIATE LIGAMENT INJURIES

What It Is

? Doctors in the United States see nearly 100,000 tears of the anterior cruciate ligament (ACL) a year and perform surgery on about half that number. Fortunately, the surgery is successful about 90% of the time.

The ACL keeps the knee stabilized by preventing the leg bone (tibia) from sliding forward beneath the thighbone (femur) during twisting and pivoting movements (see figure). ACL tears most often occur in young people (ages 15 to 25) who participate in sports such as soccer, basketball, and volleyball. These sports require players to make sudden stops when running, or jump and pivot a lot. Athletes who wear shoes with cleats and skiers—who have to change direction or twist rapidly—are also prime candidates for ACL injuries. Direct contact, such as in a football tackle, can tear the ligament, too.

When it comes to ACL injuries, there is a big gender gap (see box, p 171). Studies show teenage girls and young women are several times more likely to suffer an ACL tear than their male counterparts in the same sport. The overall increase in ACL injuries in recent years is partly attributed to the large influx of girls into sports. There are many theories about why women are vulnerable to ACL injuries, but more research is needed to pinpoint the causes.

Signs and Symptoms

An injury to the ACL usually produces immediate pain, but frequently the pain subsides quickly. You may hear a "pop" and feel your knee give way when you try to put weight on it. Within a few hours, the knee usually will swell and may hurt if you stand on it.

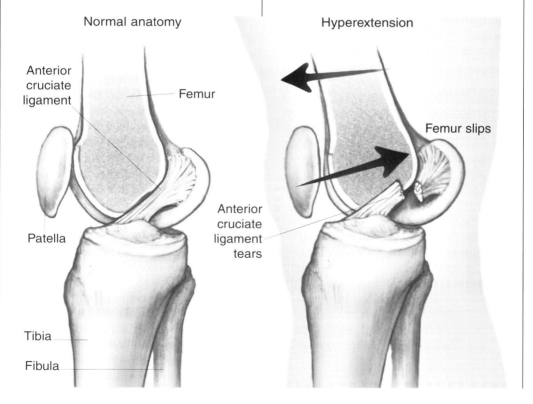

Normal anatomy

Anterior cruciate ligament

Femur

Patella

Anterior cruciate ligament tears

Tibia

Fibula

Hyperextension

Femur slips

When to Call the Doctor

If you have these symptoms, you need to be seen by a doctor for a diagnosis. In the meantime, you should apply ice to control the swelling and keep the knee elevated. Take an anti-inflammatory pain reliever such as ibuprofen. Don't walk or run on the knee since that can lead to further knee damage.

The doctor will may order an X-ray or MRI to determine the extent of the damage. In a few cases, arthroscopic inspection is necessary. This procedure is invasive, but it involves making only two tiny incisions and use of small fiber-optic instruments so the doctor can view the inside of the knee.

How to Treat It

If the ligament is only partially torn, nonsurgical treatment may be enough. A complete tear, however, usually requires surgical reconstruction, especially if you are a younger athlete who wants to return to your chosen sport. However, if you are older and not very active and your overall knee stability seems good, the doctor may recommend a muscle strengthening program. You may also need to wear a brace and use crutches initially to provide extra stability during the healing process.

Surgical reconstruction involves replacing the torn ligament with strong, healthy tissue from another part of the knee such as a strip of tendon from the knee (the patellar tendon) or from a hamstring muscle. This tissue is passed through the inside of the joint and secured to the femur and tibia. To do this, the surgeon uses a combination of arthroscopic techniques—small incisions and a tiny camera—and larger incisions. The procedure is performed either with a general anesthetic or a regional one such as an epidural, an injection in the spinal area to numb the lower part of the body while allowing the patient to remain awake.

A lengthy rehabilitation program follows to exercise the muscles and restore the joint's strength and mobility. The process is lengthy because the exercise must be started very gradually so as not to damage the surgical repair. Initially, a physical therapist will help you with the exercises until you are able to do them at home and progress at a safe pace. You don't need fancy equipment. Your doctor may recommend that you wear a knee brace for a while after surgery, and you may not be able to return to your sport for 6 months to a year. Continuing with exercises to strengthen the calf and thigh muscles can help prevent a recurrence.

:::

ACL Injuries: A True Gender Gap

The incidence of ACL injuries among female basketball players is twice that for male players. Female soccer players have four times as many ACL injuries as their male counterparts. So why the gender gap?

There are several theories, but doctors don't yet know for sure. It's probably a combination of factors related to differences between female and male anatomy, hormones, and brain/muscle interaction. Research is ongoing to determine both the causes and possible solutions. Meanwhile, a number of high school and college sports programs have instituted highly successful knee injury prevention programs that teach female athletes how to build up their leg muscles to better protect their knees and how to safely land and pivot. See the AAOS website (www.aaos.org) for more information about research in this area.

:::

Prevention

✔ Young athletes who participate in high-risk sports, as described above, should learn to land safely from a jump. With knees bent, you should land on the ball of the foot, then rock back to the middle of the foot. You can also practice cutting maneuvers by learning to pivot in a crouched rather than an upright position. Instead of coming to a stop with one big step, try three little ones, keeping the knees bent. These are motor skills that should be taught early and can be practiced and improved on.

Exercises such as leg presses and squats to strengthen your legs are important, too. Talk to your coach, athletic trainer, or doctor about a program of leg strengthening exercises that's right for you.

Don't neglect muscle conditioning and skills drills until just before the sports season starts. Make it a year-round effort.

POSTERIOR CRUCIATE LIGAMENT TEAR

What It Is

❓ The posterior cruciate ligament (PCL) is located in the back of the knee and works with the ACL in the front to connect the thighbone (femur) and the leg bone (tibia). The PCL prevents the tibia from moving too

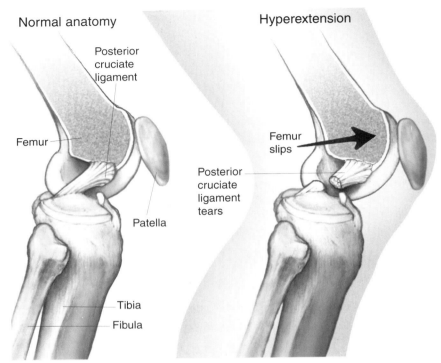

Normal anatomy

Posterior cruciate ligament

Femur

Patella

Tibia

Fibula

Hyperextension

Femur slips

Posterior cruciate ligament tears

far backward. It is considered to be the strongest knee ligament and doesn't tear as easily as the ACL, but it will if the knee is hit with sufficient impact such as

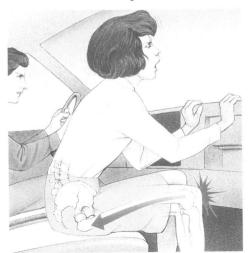

when football or soccer players land forcefully with their bent knees. Sometimes it happens when a driver or passenger's bent knee strikes the dashboard during a motor vehicle accident or a pedestrian slips on ice and lands on the knee.

PCL injuries are categorized as either isolated or combined. Isolated injuries—either partial or complete tears—don't involve any other structures in the knee and can usually be treated without surgery. Combined PCL injuries involve other ligaments, bone, nerves, or blood vessels. A dislocated knee, for example, might damage the PCL along with several other knee structures.

Signs and Symptoms

Often, the symptoms are minimal. There may be slight swelling and some pain in the back of the knee. It will hurt more when you move your knee, and you may find it difficult to walk. Your knee may feel unstable, as if it's going to give way.

When to Call the Doctor

If you've suffered an injury and your knee is showing the signs described above, call the doctor. An MRI (magnetic resonance image) can usually confirm the diagnosis. An X-ray won't show ligaments but can show if the PCL has pulled off a piece of the bone with it when it tore. If so, you have what's called an avulsion fracture of the bone.

How to Treat It

If you have an isolated and minor PCL tear, the treatment is RICE (rest, ice, compression, and elevation). Your doctor will tell you to stay off your feet or use crutches, apply ice 20 minutes two or three times a day, wrap your knee with an elastic bandage, and keep your knee propped up on pillows or otherwise elevated when you are sitting or lying down.

You can also take an anti-inflammatory medication such as ibuprofen for the pain for up to several weeks. Once the swelling goes down, the doctor will recommend a rehabilitation program to strengthen your muscles and restore your knee's range of motion. You might also need to wear a brace if you resume playing contact sports.

For more complex injuries, surgery may be necessary to stabilize the knee. Repair of an avulsion fracture sometimes requires insertion of internal screws to hold the bone in place while it heals. A complete tear may have to be reconstructed using a graft from another tendon, usually the patellar tendon, or the hamstring muscle. After the surgery, you'll probably have to use crutches or a knee brace until your strength returns and you can walk comfortably. You'll also receive instruction from a physical therapist on exercises to increase the strength of your leg muscles, especially the hamstrings. Full recovery can take up to a year.

Prevention

Unfortunately, even in well-conditioned athletes, a fall can lead to a PCL injury.

MEDIAL AND LATERAL COLLATERAL LIGAMENT INJURIES

What It Is

The medial collateral ligament (MCL) can be injured alone or in combination with the anterior cruciate (ACL). The lateral collateral ligament (LCL) is the least frequently injured of the major knee ligaments. The word lateral means side, and that's where these two structures are, with the medial on the inside of the knee and the lateral on the outside.

The MCL can be injured if the outside of the knee takes a direct blow that stretches the ligament on the inside. This sometimes happens in contact sports such as football or hockey. The LCL could be hurt by a blow to the outside of the knee.

Signs and Symptoms

With a collateral ligament injury, you may hear a pop or a crack and your knee may buckle sideways. Pain and swelling are typical, too.

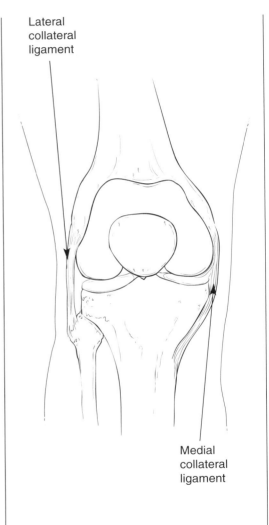

Lateral collateral ligament

Medial collateral ligament

When to Call the Doctor

If your knee is swollen and painful following an injury, it's best to see a doctor to have it evaluated. The problem may be minor and need only simple treatment such as wearing a brace until it heals. If ligament injuries are not treated properly and promptly, however, they can lead to chronic instability and many more problems later.

How to Treat It

If you have to wait for an appointment with your doctor, you should wrap your knee in an elastic bandage, keep your leg elevated as much as possible, and apply an ice pack 15 to 20 minutes four to six times a day. Take an anti-inflammatory medication such as ibuprofen to relieve pain.

The doctor may recommend that you wear a sleeve-like brace to support the knee while it heals, a process that could take a few weeks. When the pain and swelling are gone, the doctor will recommend a rehabilitation program of exercises to strengthen the muscles and restore range of motion.

If the tear is severe or is accompanied by an ACL injury, you'll probably need surgery to repair it.

Is It An Emergency?

If you can move your foot and ankle freely following a knee injury and have no numbness in your leg, and if your leg is not deformed except for some swelling, you probably don't have to rush to the emergency room. But if you have to wait a few days to visit your doctor and your knee hurts if you walk on it, use a pair of crutches.

Prevention

Prevent knee injuries by getting into shape before you start playing a sport. Several months ahead, begin a conditioning program that not only strengthens and stretches the muscles of your lower extremities and trunk but also increases your cardiovascular fitness by incorporating aerobic exercise (biking, swimming, walking, etc) for 15 to 20 minutes three to four times a week. Also, under the direction of a coach or athletic trainer, begin some agility drills that teach you cutting, jumping, and running patterns using proper form.

ADOLESCENT KNEE PAIN

What It Is

? Today's athletic adolescents, especially girls, sometimes find chronic knee pain is slowing them down. Several parts of the knee can be the source of the pain, but usually there is one underlying cause—overuse. The adolescent may be playing too long or hard, not stretching leg muscles before vigorous activity, or not wearing shoes that provide proper support, for example.

A direct hit—on or off the playing field—can lead to knee pain, too. Occasionally, the cause is not activity related. Bones that aren't aligned properly have a harder time supporting the body. Being born with knock-knees, for example, or an abnormal hip rotation can sometimes lead to knee pain years later.

Osgood-Schlatter disease (See p 198 for more information.) is one cause of knee pain in children. Other painful conditions in active adolescents include iliotibial band syndrome (See p 162 for more information.) and chondromalacia, which develops as the cartilage under the kneecap softens and causes mild pain and "grinding" sounds.

Patellofemoral pain syndrome refers to an array of problems that all produce one key symptom: aching pain along the sides of the kneecap. This is very common in girls and is due to the changing body at the hips and pelvis, which, in turn, changes the mechanics of the kneecap. The treatment of these problems is similar.

Signs and Symptoms

Usually, a dull pain develops gradually (unless the knee has suffered a direct blow) under and around the kneecap. The pain may flare up when you run, jump, climb, squat, or participate in other activities that involve repeatedly bending the knee. In some cases, the knee may be swollen or tender to touch, and you may hear a popping sound when you climb stairs or stand up after sitting for a long time. If left untreated, the knee may start to buckle or give way from the pain.

How to Treat It

Stop the activities that you suspect have caused the pain and rest your knee until it has time to heal. If it's swollen, apply an ice pack or ice wrapped in a towel for 20 minutes, two to three times a day until the swelling goes down. You can also take anti-inflammatory medications such as ibuprofen for pain relief. It may be helpful to give your knee extra support while it heals with a knee sleeve with a hole cut out for the kneecap. You can buy one in a sporting goods store. Make sure it's long enough to extend a few inches above and below the knee (approximately 8" to 12" in total length).

After symptoms disappear, return to your sport gradually. Also, build up the strength and flexibility of your thigh muscles—quadriceps and hamstrings—with exercises specifically for those areas. Or try cross training with swimming, bike riding, a cross-country ski machine or other activities that stretch and strengthen the leg muscles.

. . . .

When to Call the Doctor

If the pain persists for more than 48 hours or prevents you from bearing weight on your leg, call the doctor.

Along with an examination of the knee, the doctor may order X-rays to aid in diagnosis. Recommended treatments, aside from the ones listed above, may include a knee brace, customized shoe inserts, and a rehabilitation program with a physical therapist.

If these treatments don't solve the problem, the doctor may perform arthroscopic surgery to remove cartilage fragments and make other repairs. (See p 187 for a description of arthroscopic surgery.)

Prevention

If you are overweight, lose some pounds. Make sure your shoes are providing proper support. (See p 234 for buying advice.) Warm up with stretching exercises before beginning physical activity and stop if your knee hurts. Avoid overtraining for your sport. If, for example, you run competitively, limit the miles you run when you train or compete.

BOW LEGS

What It Is

Do your toddler's legs bow out at the knees? Or perhaps your child's knees

bump together, a condition often called knock-knees. If so, don't worry.

It's actually quite common and normal for the legs of 1- and 2-year olds to bow when they first start walking. In some children, it's quite dramatic but still normal. The knock-kneed look is more common in 3- to 6-year olds. By the time children get to be adolescents, they will grow out of it and their legs will straighten out and look normal or close to it. Neither of these conditions causes pain or other symptoms.

How to Treat It

Let nature take its course. Corrective shoes or braces that might have been considered in the past are not necessary and can actually hinder the child's walk, not to mention causing embarrassment.

When to Call the Doctor

Pediatricians evaluate children's development during regular checkups, and you should always feel free to ask questions about any specific concerns you have during those office visits. Don't wait, however, for the next visit if you suspect a more serious problem or if your child complains of discomfort. In rare cases, these conditions can be caused by an infection, arthritis, or other problems. Call, for example, if only one leg is affected, if the child is limping, or if the problem seems to get worse instead of better after the age when it would normally be expected to start improving.

CARTILAGE TEARS

What It Is

One of the most common knee injuries is to the cartilage (menisci), two wedge-shaped cushions of rubbery tissue that lie on either side of the knee joint. The cartilage pads lie freely in the joint, attached only to the side of it by the joint lining (capsule). They help provide stability for the joint and extra padding for the knee. They are, in effect, the knee's shock absorbers.

Tearing this cartilage is a common injury in football and other contact sports, especially from a tackle. The injury also can happen if you pivot or twist the upper part of your leg while your foot stays in place, a common move in tennis or basketball. Often, it happens in combination with other injuries such as an anterior cruciate ligament (ACL) tear. But athletes aren't the only ones who are vulnerable.

If you are older, your knee cartilage has weakened and thinned over the years. You may experience a cartilage tear without any particular trauma. It can happen if you merely stand up after being in a squatting position while gardening or if you twist awkwardly when you rise from a chair. Sometimes the meniscus tears from repetitive force such as happens when you run.

Signs and Symptoms

You might hear or feel a popping sensation in the joint and feel mild pain, especially when you straighten your knee. Usually you'll still be able to walk on the knee, and some athletes continue playing on it (although this is not usually a good idea!). Gradually over a 2- to 3-day period, the knee becomes stiff and swollen.

You may also notice that the knee feels as if it is locking, catching, or giving way. The pain typically is centered on the inside or outside of the knee, especially if you twist or squat. The pain and other symptoms tend to wax and wane, depending on your activity level, rather than remain constant.

When to Call the Doctor

If your knee shows no improvement after a week or so of home treatment, or if it isn't back to normal in a few weeks, or if the symptoms are severe, see your doctor as these signs could indicate a tear. Without treatment, a cartilage fragment may loosen and drift into the knee joint, causing it to lock in position so you can't bend or straighten it. At that point, you may only be able to move your knee with your hands.

Diagnostic tests may include an X-ray or an MRI. In more complex cases, such as when the knee locks, the doctor may have to reach a diagnosis by inserting an arthroscope—a fiber-optic camera connected to a monitor—through an tiny incision to view the inside of the knee.

How to Treat It

When symptoms first appear, you can't tell whether the cartilage is merely irritated or torn. If it's an irritation, you may be able to treat it successfully at home, provided the pain is tolerable and your knee still has most of its range of motion. Decrease activity so your knee can rest, apply ice packs, and take anti-inflammatory medication such as ibuprofen to relieve pain. Minimize walking, twisting, or squatting. If your symptoms improve, do some exercises to strengthen the muscles around the joint and slowly return to your normal activities.

Cartilage tears can be treated without surgery if there are no mechanical problems such as locking, if the knee is not so irritated that it is making fluid, and if the tear is small, such as in the case of an older person whose cartilage degenerates from wear. RICE (rest, ice, compression, and elevation) is the standard initial treatment.

The doctor is likely to prescribe the following:

1. Rest the knee or use crutches when you walk.

2. Apply ice packs for 20 minutes two or three times a day to reduce swelling. This can be done for 2 to 3 weeks, as necessary. Wrap the knee snugly (but not so tightly that it causes pain or ankle swelling, which could be a sign that circulation is being restricted) in an elastic compression bandage.

3. Elevate your knee as much as possible. Prop it up on pillows when you sit or recline.

4. Take an anti-inflammatory medication such as ibuprofen to relieve the pain.

5. Follow a prescribed exercise program to strengthen the muscles around the joint.

If your cartilage tear continues to produce symptoms, you may need surgery to repair it, using an arthroscope and instruments inserted in small incisions. Afterward, you'll have to undergo rehabilitation exercises until the knee's strength returns, typically from 3 to 6 weeks.

Doctors tend to treat young athletes with significant cartilage tears aggressively. Surgical repair makes it more likely that they will be able to return to their sport.

Prevention

 Even in well-conditioned athletes, this isn't an injury that's preventable.

GROWING PAINS

What It Is

? Some people think they are a myth, but parents whose children have experienced unexplained leg pain will tell you growing pains are real. Although the cause isn't known, doctors think the condition is probably related to muscle stress from overactivity such as running, jumping, and climbing. A particularly active day sometimes leads to aching legs at night. It's a fairly common occurrence and not cause for concern.

Growing pains is a misnomer in that there isn't any evidence linking the pain to growing bones. It seems to be more common in boys than in girls, and it most often affects children ages 2 to 5 years but also affects children in the 8- to 12-year age range.

Signs and Symptoms

The child complains of pain in the late afternoon or evening but has no visible signs of injury. Sometimes kids wake up crying at night. The pain is usually felt primarily in the calf or thigh, but some children also report pain in the foot, ankle, or knee. Often the pain is in both legs, but one may hurt more than the other or one may hurt one night and the other hurt another night. Usually the pain is intermittent in that it only occurs occasionally, not daily. With all these variations, it's no wonder some parents think their kids are faking or imagining their pain! Perhaps the most telling sign of

What About Heel Pain After Play?

Sometimes children have heel pain and a slight limp after active play or sports. This may be mistaken for growing pains but is actually the result of stress to the calcaneal apophysis, which is the part of the heel bone that hasn't grown together (fused) in the still-growing child. Therefore, the heel is susceptible to overuse injury. This condition, sometimes called Sever disease (even though it isn't a disease), usually affects girls younger than age 9 and boys younger than age 11. After that, the bone fuses and the potential for the problem disappears. Usually the only treatment needed is for the child to ease up on the activity that caused the pain. For prompt pain relief, the child should rest the foot, apply ice packs for 15 to 20 minutes three or four times a day, and take over-the-counter anti-inflammatory medications such as ibuprofen.

growing pains is if the child has had a particularly active day before complaining of the pain.

How to Treat It

Many parents find that massaging the legs and cuddling their children provides relief (or at least a distraction!). You can also try hot or cold compresses. If your child seems especially uncomfortable, you can also give him the pain reliever your pediatrician normally recommends and remind him that he'll outgrow the problem eventually.

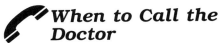

When to Call the Doctor

With growing pains, children usually like to be massaged. If the child has an actual injury, the leg will hurt when touched. If the latter is the case or if your child limps, has a fever, or other signs of illness or if part of the leg is swollen, red, or persistently painful, call your doctor. These are signs of other conditions that need prompt treatment. The way doctors diagnose the pain in these instances is by ruling out other possible causes.

JUMPER'S KNEE

What It Is

Tendons are the tough bands that connect muscles to bones. But sometimes they aren't tough enough. Tendinitis (inflammation) or a torn (ruptured) tendon can develop if you put too much stress on the knee with a variety of activities, especially jumping. Kneecap (patellar) tendinitis is sometimes called jumper's knee. During a jump, the quadriceps muscles (the big ones in front of your thigh) may contract too far and overstretch the quadriceps tendon above the kneecap or the patellar tendon below it (see figure). This can occur in basketball and vol-

leyball, and it often happens to people who aren't in good condition when they get into the game. Older people whose tendons are weaker can get tendinitis from lifting something heavy.

Signs and Symptoms

Pain in the front of the knee is the key symptom of tendinitis. You can usually feel a tender spot where the pain is concentrated. It may be more noticeable right after you exercise or if you sit, squat, or kneel for long periods. Activity, such as climbing stairs or running, makes the pain worse. If the tendon actually tears (ruptures), you'll not only have acute pain but you won't be able to straighten your knee, lift your leg, or stand on it.

How to Treat It

 If you have symptoms of tendinitis, stop the activity that aggravated your knee so it can rest and recuperate. Keep it elevated as much as practical for the first few days and apply ice for 20 minutes, two or three times a day. Take an anti-inflammatory medication such as ibuprofen to relieve the pain.

- -

When to Call the Doctor

Call if your symptoms fit the description of a tendon tear or if your symptoms of tendinitis don't improve in 5 to 7 days, despite treatment or if the symptoms worsen. You may need an MRI so the doctor can identify a partial or complete tear of the tendon. If there is a complete tear, you'll need surgery to reattach the ends, and you'll have to wear a cast or a brace and use crutches for 3 to 6 weeks. If the tendon is only partially torn, you'll wear a knee brace for approximately 3 to 4 weeks to immobilize the knee while it heals.

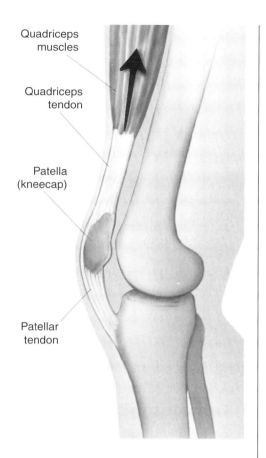

Quadriceps muscles

Quadriceps tendon

Patella (kneecap)

Patellar tendon

In either case, you'll need physical therapy to rehabilitate the knee. This involves exercises to restore flexibility and strengthen the quadriceps and hamstring muscles. Other physical therapy treatments, such as ultrasound, may also be recommended. Ultrasound uses gentle sound waves to increase the circulation of blood to the injured area. It is applied by the therapist using a small wand-like instrument that is rubbed over the injury site.

Later, as you resume your normal activities, you may find it helpful to support your knee by wearing a sleeve or a compression strap around the injured tendon. As you gradually return to activities, you'll find that applying heat before an activity and ice afterwards often is helpful. It may take as long as 6 months for rehabili-

tation to be complete, but you can probably return to many activities before that time.

Prevention

✓ Get your leg muscles into good condition before you begin a sport that involves a lot of jumping or bouncing. Don't accelerate your exercise program suddenly.

KNEE ARTHRITIS

What It Is

? When you think about the countless times you bend or put weight on your knee in just one day, it isn't surprising that over a few decades, the joint would start to wear out. One of the most common knee problems in middle-aged and older people is osteoarthritis (OA). It's sometimes called degenerative or "wear-and-tear" arthritis. The constant stress on the knee causes the cushion of cartilage between the bones to literally wear away. At that point, the bones start to rub together and, as a result, the joint can become inflamed and painful.

A second, less common type, is rheumatoid arthritis (RA), an autoimmune disease that can affect multiple joints in the body and produces symptoms similar

to OA. It usually starts at a younger age than OA, and women are three times more likely to have it than men.

A third type is post-traumatic arthritis that develops, sometimes years later, after the knee has been injured.

Signs and Symptoms

Usually the primary symptoms—pain and swelling—develop gradually, although a few people experience the pain suddenly. You're also likely to have knee stiffness and pain when you get up in the morning, but it gets better as you move around. Sometimes the knee makes a clicking sound when it is bent or straightened. You may feel weakness in the knee that leads to locking or

184

buckling. If the arthritis is severe, you may even have pain that wakes you up at night.

When to Call the Doctor

It's best to consult your doctor when you have these symptoms to rule out other conditions with similar signs and determine which type of arthritis you have. Diagnostic tests may include X-rays, which can show loss of joint space. Diagnosing RA may require blood tests.

How to Treat It

Lifestyle changes may be all the treatment you need, at least in the early stages. You can minimize the activities that aggravate your knees, switching, for example, from jogging to swimming for exercise. If you are overweight, shed some pounds to lighten the load on the knees. You might also try wearing a knee brace or knee sleeve and energy-absorbing shoes. Your doctor may recommend applying ice or liniments, both of which can provide temporary relief from the aching and stiffness. Some people with arthritis benefit from using a cane while walking.

Several types of medications are used to treat knee arthritis. For mild symptoms, over-the-counter anti-inflammatory pain relievers often work. For more serious

Exercise Without Stress

For people who love cycling, recumbent bicycles offer a way for arthritis sufferers to get exercise without adding much stress to the knee. Riders of recumbent bikes sit lower to the ground, perched on a seat with a back instead of a saddle. These bikes are easier and more comfortable to peddle, but they aren't designed for speed or hilly terrain.

Water exercises are also excellent for arthritis sufferers. The water soothes the aching joint while the exercises help strengthen the supportive muscles.

pain, your doctor may prescribe an oral medication or corticosteroid injections into the knee. Preliminary evidence shows that glucosamine and chondroitin sulfate may be helpful in relieving symptoms and delaying the progression of OA in the knee. A large research study funded by the National Institutes of Health (NIH) currently is underway to evaluate the effectiveness of these supplements. Results are expected to be published in 2005. The NIH is also studying the effectiveness of acupuncture and magnets in relieving the symptoms of OA.

When other measures fail, you may need arthroscopic surgery, which uses pencil-thin fiber optic instruments inserted in tiny incisions. People whose functioning has become severely limited may opt for a total knee replacement. (See below to learn more about this procedure.)

Prevention

Doctors don't yet know how to prevent RA. You may be able to head off OA by avoiding overstressing your knees. Start exercising gradually and keep your leg muscles toned with exercises to improve strength and flexibility. Wear comfortable, supportive shoes to prevent knee as well as foot problems. (See p 234 for buying advice.) If you have a knee injury, seek treatment promptly and follow your doctor's advice to avoid posttraumatic arthritis later.

KNEE REPLACEMENT SURGERY

The past 20 years have seen dramatic advances in techniques to treat knee injuries. And a good thing, too. Baby boomers who are remaining physically active into their later years, coupled with longer life expectancy in general, will only increase the number of knee joints that will wear out before their owners do.

One of the most important of these treatments is the use of artificial joints to replace "native" joints that have been damaged by wear and tear. The procedure is called knee replacement surgery or total knee arthroplasty (TKA). The goal is to eliminate pain so that you can resume most normal activities. People with artificial knees can hike, bike, and play

Knees Go First

More joint replacements are performed on knees than on any other joint in the body. Orthopaedic surgeons perform knee replacement procedures on 400,000 knees a year with a high rate of success. But just as with real knees, artificial joints can wear out. Approximately 95% of knee replacements last 15 to 20 years. After that, a patient may need a second (revision) surgery.

tennis or golf, for example. They just have to avoid certain activities that can overstress the joint.

What It Is

? Knee replacement surgery is recommended for people who are experiencing severe pain and disability due to osteoarthritis (OA), rheumatoid arthritis (RA), or trauma. Often, these patients have already undergone arthroscopic surgery for pain relief. Arthroscopy is a less invasive procedure than knee replacement and can remove torn cartilage and other debris and make repairs. This is done through tiny incisions that accommodate pencil-sized surgical instruments and a fiber-optic camera that projects a picture on a video screen to guide the surgeon. Unfortunately, arthroscopic surgery may not solve the problem forever. Then your doctor may recommend knee replacement.

Several weeks before surgery, you may want to donate blood that can later be used during the surgery if you need a transfusion. This is called autotransfusion. Usually patients also make a pre-operative visit to the hospital. During that visit, you may undergo tests such as X-rays, a blood test, and urinalysis. You'll be given instructions on how to prepare for the operation, such as fasting after midnight before your surgery. Your doctor also may advise you to stop taking some medications such as aspirin, ibuprofen, or herbals and supplements prior to surgery. Make sure

Ask Your Surgeon About the Video

Some surgeons have videotapes you can watch that give you a detailed description of knee replacement surgery and recovery. Ask yours if there is one available.

you tell your doctor early on if you are taking any kind of medication.

This is the time to ask any questions that you still have about the type of anesthesia to be used, what to expect during your recovery period in the hospital, and anything else you're still wondering about. When you are admitted to the hospital and prior to your surgery, the knee that is to be operated on will be marked with special ink so there can be no mix-up in the operating room.

What Is a Prosthesis?

In a total knee arthroplasty (TKA), the worn out cartilage surfaces of the bones of the joint are replaced by a prosthesis (sometimes called an implant) made of metal alloys, high-grade plastics, or other construction materials. Most of the other parts of the knee, such as the ligaments that connect the bones, remain intact.

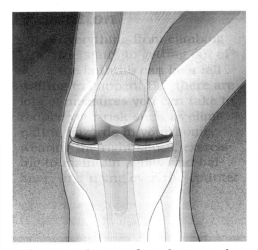

The actual type of implant used and its expected longevity depend on such factors as your age, weight, activity level, and general health. There are more than 150 knee replacement designs on the market today from several manufacturers. Your surgeon will discuss with you what type will be used in your procedure. You'll be allowed to handle a sample of the prosthesis if you care to. A prosthesis simulates your natural knee as much as possible, and after you heal from the surgery you shouldn't notice it is there. Prostheses weigh only a few ounces, they rarely make a noise when they move, and although they contain metal, they don't rust.

If both of your knees need replacing, your doctor may recommend you have them done at separate times. That way, you have one good leg to stand on, with the help of crutches or a walker, while the other recovers.

How Knee Replacement Surgery Is Done

Knee replacement is major surgery and is done in a hospital with general anesthesia. Before the implant can be placed in the knee, the surgeon makes an incision between 6" and 12" long, usually lengthwise through the front of the knee just to the side of the kneecap. Through the incision, the surgeon moves the kneecap and muscles to the side and removes the pieces of cartilage between the two leg bones that form the joint. Often the tissue under the kneecap is also removed. Then the surgeon cements the prosthesis into place. If any ligaments have contracted due to pain and deformity before surgery, the surgeon releases them so they'll function as close to normal as possible.

What to Expect After Surgery

Pain following the procedure varies from person to person but can be controlled with medication. You are typically in the hospital for 3 to 7 days depending on how fast you heal. Frequently you are given the opportunity before surgery to learn what you will need to do to promote healing when you are discharged from the hospital.

Usually, your physical therapy starts the day after your surgery. The physical therapist will help

....

Passing the Metal Detector

Although your prosthesis doesn't have enough metal in it to set off most airport security alarms, the sensitivity of these machines can vary. Your surgeon can give you a Medic-Alert card attesting to your knee replacement, should you ever need one to show security guards.

....

you bend and straighten your knee and will also teach you how to exercise to regain the strength and range of motion in your leg once you get home. You'll also be taught how to care for the incision and how to modify your normal activities until you regain the full use of your knee.

Modifying Activities After Surgery

1. Rearrange your furniture so you can navigate easily with crutches.

2. Avoid going up and down stairs at first, which may mean moving your bed.

3. Consider modifications to your bathroom, such as adding a shower chair, grab bars, and a raised toilet seat.

4. Remove throw rugs or extension cords that might cause you to slip and fall.

5. Use assistive devices such as a long-handled shoehorn and a grabbing tool to pick things up so you don't have to bend too far.

If your right knee was replaced, you should avoid driving for 6 to 8 weeks. With a left knee replacement, you may be able to drive a week after returning home if your car has an automatic transmission. It may be 6 to 8 weeks before you can return to work, depending on your job requirements. Sexual relations can be resumed 4 to 6 weeks after surgery.

Osteotomy and Unicompartmental Arthroplasty

If you have early-stage arthritis and the damage is limited to one part of the knee, your surgeon may recommend one of two other procedures to relieve your pain.

An osteotomy (cutting of the bone) is sometimes recommended for people younger than age 60 or who are very active. With this procedure, the surgeon reshapes the shinbone (tibia) or thighbone (femur), realigning the healthy bone and cartilage to compensate for the damaged tissue. When the joint alignment is repositioned away from the damaged area, your knee can glide freely and carry weight evenly. After surgery, your knee will be held in place with a cast, staples, or internal plate devices. Depending on how fast you heal, you'll be on crutches for 1 to 3 months, and following rehabilitation, should be able to resume regular activities after 3 to 6 months.

One drawback of osteotomy is that your knee may not look symmetrical afterward. This happens if you are bow-legged or knock-kneed and only one of your knee joints requires surgical correction. Also, you may still need a TKA some day, which can be more technically challenging for the surgeon if you've already had an osteotomy. This is because some of the bone is removed in the first procedure, leaving less for the surgeon to work with in the second one.

Unicompartmental knee arthroplasty (UKA) is sometimes recommended for people older than age 60 who are relatively sedentary but not obese. The recovery period is shorter than with TKA or osteotomy. If you have arthritis in only one side of your knee, then only the parts on that side need replacing rather than the entire joint, as in TKA. UKA provides better joint function because both cruciate ligaments (the major stabilizing ligaments in the knee) and other healthy parts of the knee are preserved. Compared with osteotomy, UKA has a higher initial success rate, fewer complications, and less blood loss during surgery.

Candidates for UKA surgery are screened carefully. They must not have significant inflammation, must have an intact anterior cruciate ligament (ACL), and must have damage that is confined to only one compartment of the knee. The procedure involves removal of the diseased bone and insertion of two small replacement parts. This relieves pain and delays the need for a TKA, although this might become necessary in the future.

KNEE BURSITIS

What It Is

? Bursae are fluid-filled sacs nestled between the bones and soft tissues and which provide cushioning. If the bursae become irritated, they produce too much fluid, causing them to swell and put pressure on the adjacent parts of the knee. This irritation is called bursitis.

Two common places in the knee where this happens are between the skin and the bone of the kneecap (prepatellar bursitis) and just below the knee joint (goose-foot, also called pes anserine bursitis) (see figure).

In kneecap (prepatellar) bursitis, the fluid-filled bursa forms a dome-shaped swelling on top of the kneecap. This type of bursitis is sometimes called "housemaid's knee" because it can be caused by pressure from constant kneeling. Carpet installers, plumbers, and gardeners are susceptible. The condition also can be caused by a blow to the knee during contact sports, especially football,

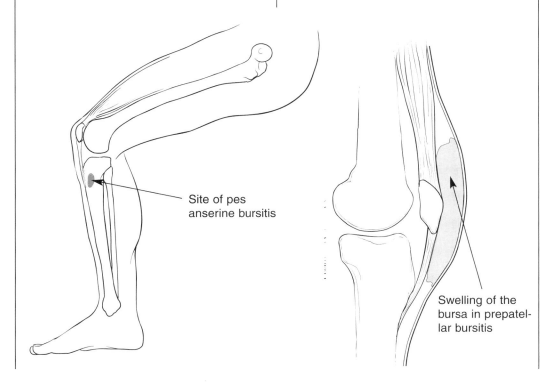

Site of pes anserine bursitis

Swelling of the bursa in prepatellar bursitis

baseball, wrestling, and basketball. Others at risk include people who have rheumatoid arthritis or gout.

Goosefoot (pes anserine) bursitis is caused by irritation of the pes anserine bursa located between the shinbone and three tendons of the hamstring muscle at the inside of the knee. Because these three tendons splay out on the front of the shinbone, they resemble a goose foot, hence the nickname. This type of bursitis is common in people with osteoarthritis or those who are obese. Runners are susceptible as well.

Signs and Symptoms

With prepatellar bursitis, rapid swelling on the front of the kneecap and pain with activity are common. There may be pain at night, too, if there is a lot of swelling. The knee will be tender and warm to the touch.

With pes anserine bursitis, pain develops slowly on the inside of the knee and sometimes in the center of the shinbone, about 2" below the knee joint. The pain is worse when you climb stairs, exercise, or otherwise put stress on the hamstring muscles where they connect with the leg bone (tibia).

How to Treat It

As long as the bursa is merely inflamed and not infected, you can probably treat it effectively yourself. Treatment is the same for both types of bursitis. Stop doing the activity that caused the pain until the condition clears up. To reduce the swelling, apply an ice pack at regular intervals three or four times a day for 20 minutes at a time. You should notice a reduction in the swelling after each icing session, as long as you are also resting the knee. Also, keep the knee elevated as much as possible. Anti-inflammatory medication such as ibuprofen will help reduce the inflammation and ease the pain.

When to Call the Doctor

If the pain doesn't improve after a couple of days of home treatment, call the doctor. The symptoms of pes anserine bursitis can mimic a stress fracture, so an X-ray is necessary for a diagnosis.

The doctor may decide the bursa should be drained (aspirated) with a needle. The doctor will inject a small amount of anesthetic first to numb the area or spray a numbing preparation on the skin. Then the fluid is drawn out with a syringe, much like having blood drawn. This will immediately reduce the swelling. The doctor also may recommend an injection of a solution containing anesthetic and a steroid that can decrease the inflammation and produce prompt pain relief.

In chronic cases of bursitis, your doctor may recommend surgical removal of the bursa.

Prevention

✔ To prevent prepatellar bursitis, wear knee pads when working on your knees or when participating in high-risk sports. Also, if you must do a lot of kneeling, take frequent breaks to stretch your legs and switch to other activities whenever possible.

To prevent pes anserine bursitis in runners, be sure to incorporate stretching exercises into your warm-up routine, especially to loosen the hamstring muscles. When you are in training, avoid excessive hill running. Work on increasing your mileage gradually, since sudden increases can over-stress your knees.

LEG CRAMPS

What It Is

? Have you ever been awakened at night by a sharp leg cramp? This sudden painful spasm may happen to you occasionally or even frequently with no particular cause except possibly overexertion during the day. You may also get a cramp after sitting or lying in an awkward position for a long time or during sports. In most cases, it's harmless—except for the pain—and nothing to worry about.

If the cramps are accompanied by other symptoms or if the pain becomes continuous, however, you may have something more serious.

One possibility is a condition called exertional compartment syndrome (ECS). This pain is caused by prolonged running or other overtraining, which leads to excessive blood flow and causes the calf muscles to expand.

Distance runners are particularly at risk. The pain occurs in one or more of the four "compartments" in which the muscles in the lower leg are housed. Because the pain is often in the front compartment, you may be told you have anterior (front) compartment syndrome. Sometimes it happens if you switch from running on a soft surface to a hard one.

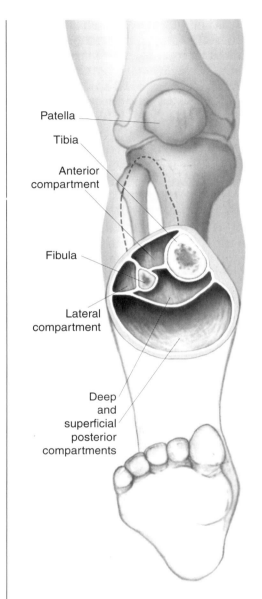

Patella
Tibia
Anterior compartment
Fibula
Lateral compartment
Deep and superficial posterior compartments

Signs and Symptoms

As you increase activity, you'll have an ache or sharp pain in your calf, often toward the front, and sometimes radiating into the foot. A few peo-ple feel a prickling or tingling feeling instead of actual pain. The pain develops gradually while you exercise but stops within 30 minutes afterwards. You won't have pain when your leg is resting.

When to Call the Doctor

Call if cramps are frequent, interfere with your physical activities, or are accompanied by other symptoms. If you have exertional compartment syndrome, an examination won't show any outward sign of problems. The way doctors diagnose it is to examine you during exercise on a treadmill, at which point the involved muscle can feel swollen, tense, and tender to touch. A needle inserted before and after the exercise session can measure the pressure change.

How to Treat It

During a cramp, your calf muscle involuntarily contracts or shortens, causing the pain. Usually you can relieve it in a few minutes by straightening your leg to stretch the muscle back out. Sometimes just standing up will do the trick, and massage may help, too.

To treat ECS initially, you'll have to stop or at least reduce the intensity of your training program to give your muscles a chance to heal. If they don't, surgery to open or free up the involved compartment may be necessary if you want to resume distance running.

Prevention

To prevent cramps, warm up properly before vigorous exercise and drink plenty of fluids. If you play a sport, incorporate conditioning exercises into your training routine to keep your muscles strong and flexible. Also, don't wear running shoes that are worn out.

LIMPING

What It Is

Most children limp at some time or another. Figuring out the reason can be a puzzle for parents and sometimes doctors, too, because there are many possible causes. Sometimes the cause is obvious—a blister on the foot or a bruised leg from a kick during a soccer game. More serious conditions that cause limping include fractures and infections in bones or joints.

When to Call the Doctor

If there was an obvious cause for the limp—such as an injury during play or sports—and your child isn't in much discomfort, you can have her rest the leg for a day or two to see if it goes away. Call immediately, however, if the limp is accompanied by a fever, swelling or redness at the joint, lethargy, or other signs of illness because this condition could be the result of an infection. Significant pain should be reported, too, as this could signal a fracture or other damage that needs prompt medical treatment.

If you don't know what the cause of the limp might be, the doctor will want to know when it started and what time of day it appears to be the worst. Typically, problems in the bones or muscles get worse the more children are active. That's why a limp from a leg or knee condition may be worse in the afternoon. A limp that is worse in the morning could be a sign of transient synovitis (temporary inflammation) in the hip (See p 163 for more information.) or childhood arthritis among other things.

Call, too, if your child is just learning to walk and you detect a limp. There are several possible

Kids Say the Darndest Things

Often a child's limp is caused by a minor injury, but you may never find out about it. A busy preschooler falls from a porch step and hurts her leg. When you notice her limping later and ask if she hurt herself, you may get a vague answer because your child really doesn't remember. So many things happen in an active child's day that falling off a step may not stand out!

causes, such as undetected congenital deformities, and the longer any of them go untreated, the harder it can be to fix.

How to Treat It

 The treatments for limping are as varied as the causes—measures as simple as

rest and ice for a sports-related knee injury to antibiotics for an infection.

Note: See the next sections in this chapter for specific conditions that can cause limping in children. (See pp 156-158 for information on pediatric hip conditions that can also cause limping.)

MUSCLE STRAIN

What It Is

A strain is a stretching or tearing of muscle fibers. It's sometimes called a pulled muscle and is a common injury to the calf (lower leg) muscle, especially during sports, weight training, or other vigorous activity. Sometimes people who haven't been active and who plunge into serious exercise without a gradual build-up will strain a muscle. Usually, a strain is easy to recov-er from with no lasting damage. (See p 159 for information on thigh muscle strains.)

Signs and Symptoms

If it's a mild strain (what doctors call a first-degree strain), you may not feel any pain until the next day, and even then it's usually mild. A more severe strain (second degree) causes a stabbing pain as soon as the injury occurs. Your calf may become stiff, swollen, and tender to touch. You're also likely to notice a bruise over the area within 24 hours, and you may not be able to walk normally. A third-degree strain is a complete separation of the muscle fibers in which case you will have severe pain and not be able to bear weight.

How to Treat It

When a muscle injury occurs, stop whatever activity you are doing. Rest the leg for a few days. Don't walk on it more than necessary. Apply an ice pack to the muscle for 20 minutes two to three times a day to reduce the swelling and pain. Wrap the area with an elastic bandage to provide compression. Don't wrap too tightly, however, because additional swelling could inhibit blood flow. Keep your leg elevated as much as possible to minimize bleeding and swelling. Don't return to your sport or exercise program until the symptoms are gone, and the joints above and below the injured muscle move without pain. Acupuncture can help reduce swelling, allowing earlier return to function.

When is a Strain a Sprain?

Doctors use the word "strain" to apply to the stretching or tearing of a muscle. The word "sprain" describes the same type of injury but to a ligament.

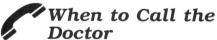

When to Call the Doctor

See your doctor if you have severe pain, numbness or difficulty moving your leg, or if your home treatment measures don't help within a few days. Call also if you have considerable swelling because this can impede blood flow without immediate medical treatment, which is potentially dangerous. When the symptoms subside, you'll probably need physical therapy to restore the muscle's flexibility and strength. If the muscle is ruptured, surgery may be necessary to repair it.

Prevention

Be sure to warm up your leg muscles before engaging in physical activity. Keep your muscles strong and flexible through exercise.

OSGOOD-SCHLATTER DISEASE

What It Is

? This is a long name for a condition (knee pain)—not a disease—that occurs in young adolescents. Fortunately, it usually heals with rest and with little or no lasting effects.

What happens is that the ends of the child's leg bones that join at the knee haven't fully hardened while the child is still growing. This makes the bones more vulnerable to tugging from muscles and tendons, especially during vigorous activity or competitive sports. During a growth spurt, the bones can also grow faster than the muscles, causing even more pulling on the joint. The outcome is that, because of the activity, the tendon of the kneecap (patellar tendon) becomes inflamed where it attaches to the shinbone (tibia). In the worst cases, the tendon may tear away and pull a tiny piece of shinbone with it.

Boys are affected more often than girls, but in girls it appears at a younger age. Boys between the ages of 10 and 15 who play sports involving a lot of running and jumping are prime candidates for Osgood-Schlatter disease.

Note: *Other conditions can cause knee pain in adolescents, too. Read the sections on the following pages to see if those symptoms fit your child's more closely.*

Signs and Symptoms

In Osgood-Schlatter disease, your child feels pain just below the knee that gets worse when he's running, jumping, or kneeling and that may go away when he rests. His knee also may hurt if he sits for long periods with the knee bent. Sometimes there is a bony bump just below the kneecap (patella) that hurts when you press on it. Occasionally, the condition exists in both knees, but, in that case, the symptoms tend to be more pronounced in one of them.

How to Treat It

The most important treatment is resting the knee. If your child complains of knee pain, don't let him play the sport that caused the overuse injury. Wait until the knee is better, then work back up to participation in the sport gradually. Other simple steps your child can take at home include applying ice to reduce inflammation and taking anti-inflammatory drugs such as ibuprofen to relieve the pain. Wearing a protective kneepad, sometimes called a knee sleeve, during physical activity may help your child get back in the game faster.

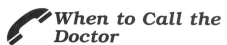

When to Call the Doctor

If the symptoms aren't responding to home treatment, call your doctor. Stubborn or severe cases of this condition sometimes require the knee to be immobilized, typically with a brace that can be removed once a day for bathing and some range-of-motion exercises. The doctor may also recommend the child stop playing his sport for 2 to 3 months until the knee has healed. It can take 6 to 7 months for the child to work back to his original level of activity.

Prevention

To prevent a recurrence, your doctor may suggest some stretching and strengthening exercises.

SHIN-SPLINTS

What It Is

There's a reason that doctors advise their patients not to "overdo it" when they decide to get in shape. Inactive people who begin a running program, for example, without gradually conditioning their leg muscles are prime candidates for overuse injuries such as shin-splints.

The phrase "shin-splints" is used to describe tenderness and pain in the lower leg. The condition and what causes it aren't completely understood. But we do know that it usually develops after physical activity such as vigorous exercise or participation in sports. Overtraining can lead to inflammation in the tendons and muscles, causing pain.

Signs and Symptoms

You'll gradually notice pain, midway between your knee and your ankle, at the beginning of vigorous activity. After you've warmed up, the pain eases, but then returns later when you've finished exercising. The area will be tender to the touch and may also be swollen.

How to Treat It

Take a break from the activity that led to the pain. That's usually enough to solve the problem. You can also take an anti-inflammatory medication such as ibuprofen to relieve the symptoms. Ice massages can help too, along with wrapping or taping the area to provide extra support.

Also, wear shoes with adequate arch supports to ease symptoms and prevent recurrences. (See p 234 for buying information.) Return to your activity gradually and be sure your routine includes exercises to stretch and strengthen the leg muscles.

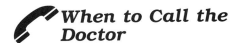

When to Call the Doctor

Pain in the lower leg that persists or increases, despite several days of home treatment, should be evaluated by your doctor.

Prevention

Start an exercise program gradually and be sure to include a warm-up and cool-down routine to keep your muscles flexible. Make sure your shoes have good arch supports and proper padding.

STRESS FRACTURES

What It Is

Exercise such as running can be good for you, but not if you overdo it. Repeated stress tires the muscles so they no longer absorb the shock. The pressure is transferred to the lower leg bones (tibia and fibula) and can cause tiny, almost invisible breaks called stress fractures. Although bones continually make new bone tissue to replace what is lost due to wear, the bone regeneration process can't keep up if the stress is unrelenting. Stress fractures that aren't given time to heal can lead to bigger cracks and more problems.

Female athletes are particularly at risk, especially those who are no longer menstruating regularly.

Signs and Symptoms

What distinguishes a stress fracture from tendinitis or other soft-tissue injuries is that you'll feel pain that becomes gradually worse the longer you exercise but improves when you rest. With soft-tissue injuries caused by overuse, the pain lessens when the muscles warm up with activity but gets worse when they cool down and tighten after vigorous exercise.

With a stress fracture, usually you won't notice any pain when you first get up in the morning. It's only after you become active that the pain starts. If you continue to exercise or play sports on the injured leg, it's likely to become swollen. The area also may be tender to the touch.

When to Call the Doctor

Call if you have pain in one area of the lower leg that increases with activity and improves with rest. If you do have a stress fracture, prompt treatment is important to prevent the crack from becoming worse.

How to Treat It

 If you take a break from running or sports so the tibia has time to regenerate, the stress fracture will heal with no lasting effects. This may take several weeks depending on the location of the injury and whether you continued to exercise on the leg after the fracture occurred. You may need to use a cane or crutches to take pressure off the

Diet Counts

Because of the high proportion of stress fractures in young female athletes, especially runners, doctors are urging them to train sensibly and also eat sensibly. Consuming adequate calcium builds strong bones and helps prevent fractures, but too many young people fall short of the recommended amount. (See p 19 for the "Healthy Bones Diet.")

leg until you can walk on it comfortably. Also, wear soft, cushioning shoes during the recovery period.

When the pain subsides, your doctor may recommend exercises to keep the muscles conditioned while the bone heals. Swimming is often recommended for maintaining overall fitness without aggravating the fracture.

Prevention

If you plan to increase the intensity or length of your workout, do so gradually.

UNSTABLE KNEECAP

What It Is

? The kneecap (patella) is usually right where it belongs—smack in front of the shinbone (tibia) and thighbone (femur) where the two come together to form the knee joint. It's there to protect the knee and give the muscles leverage. Normally the kneecap slides up or down slightly when you extend or flex your knee. Sometimes, however, it slides too far to one side or the other instead of going straight up and down (see figure, right). When this happens, such as after a sharp blow or a fall, the kneecap can partially or completely dislocate.

Dislocation is more likely to happen when the groove the kneecap is supposed to fit into is uneven or too shallow (see figure, p 203). It's also more likely if the knee joint is angled, because that's how it grew, or if your quadriceps muscle (large muscle on the front of the thigh that guides the kneecap into the groove) doesn't pull it straight. Even if you have a normal groove and muscle, the kneecap can still slip out of place if your knee receives a sharp blow, as in a fall.

Soft tissues are stretched or torn when the kneecap slips and may not return to their former length.

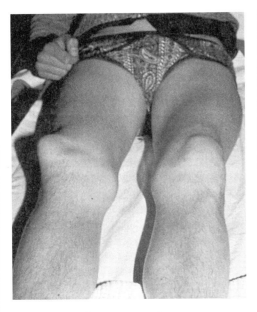

This may leave your kneecap looser than it was before the dislocation and can lead to recurrences, usually with milder symptoms than the first time but still troubling. Recurrences are also common if the original problem was that the groove your kneecap fits into isn't shaped properly or if you do not strengthen the quadriceps muscle through exercise to help it guide the kneecap correctly.

Signs and Symptoms

The severity of the symptoms depends on how far out of place the kneecap slips and how much trauma

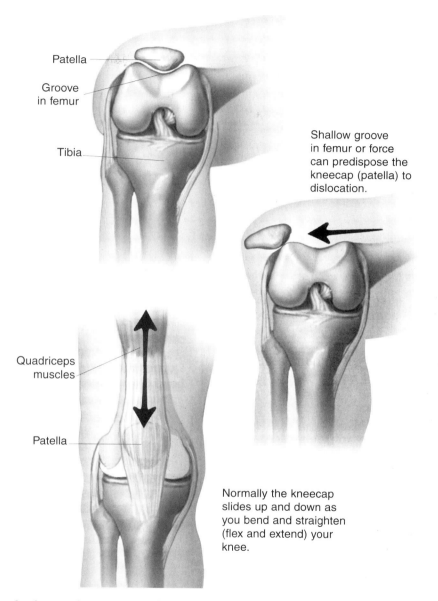

Patella

Groove
in femur

Tibia

Shallow groove
in femur or force
can predispose the
kneecap (patella) to
dislocation.

Quadriceps
muscles

Patella

Normally the kneecap
slides up and down as
you bend and straighten
(flex and extend) your
knee.

occurred when it happened. If the slip is only partial and your kneecap goes back into place by itself, you'll have acute pain, swelling, and stiffness in the front of the knee that is worse when you move around. Your knee may buckle and be unable to support your weight. You may also hear a pop when the kneecap dislocates and notice that your knee looks deformed. If it dislocates completely and remains that way, the pain will be severe, the knee will look deformed, and you won't be able to bear weight.

. . . .

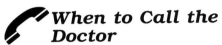

When to Call the Doctor

Any type of dislocation requires examination by a doctor. If you have the symptoms described above, go to the hospital emergency room.

How to Treat It

If your kneecap has dislocated, you will probably need pain medication to relax your muscles before the doctor can apply gentle pressure to put it back in place. Sometimes the kneecap returns to its proper position spontaneously before you reach the doctor, but you still need to be examined so the doctor can identify any other damage to your knee.

You may need to wear a brace for approximately 3 to 6 weeks until the knee tissue heals. Once the tenderness is gone, you'll be

advised to perform special exercises that strengthen the thigh muscles, especially those on the inner thigh since the kneecap usually dislocates to the outside of the groove. Cycling is often recommended as a way to build strength. If the thigh muscles are strong, they are better able to hold the kneecap in its correct position. Other types of physical therapy, including electrical stimulation, may also be recommended.

If other treatments fail to relieve the symptoms or if the problem continues to recur, surgery may be recommended.

Prevention

Always keep your thigh muscles strong and all four parts of the quadriceps muscles equally developed so that the kneecap moves up and down in its groove rather than sideways. This is especially important for girls because frequently their knees angle outward, putting them at greater risk for dislocation.

FOOT AND ANKLE

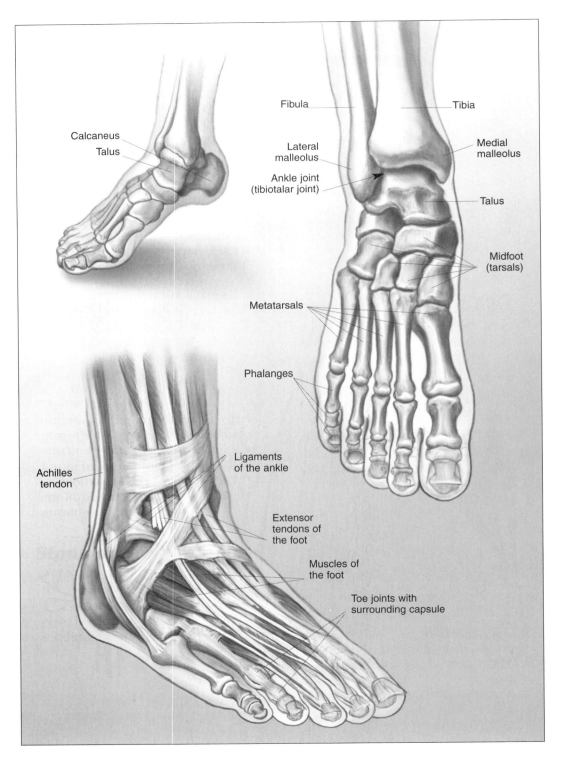

Fibula

Tibia

Calcaneus

Talus

Lateral
malleolus

Medial
malleolus

Ankle joint
(tibiotalar joint)

Talus

Midfoot
(tarsals)

Metatarsals

Phalanges

Achilles
tendon

Ligaments
of the ankle

Extensor
tendons of
the foot

Muscles of
the foot

Toe joints with
surrounding capsule

FOOT AND ANKLE

IF YOUR FEET COULD talk, they'd probably say they "Don't get no respect."

For all the things they enable us to do—walk, run, dance, climb, swim, play sports—you'd think we'd treat them better. Instead, too many people shove them into tight-fitting shoes, jog for miles on hard pavement, ignore warning signs such as calluses or pain, and don't seek treatment until foot problems become serious and harder to repair. If the feet don't work right, the legs and hips can be thrown out of balance and damaged, too.

Instead of abusing them, we should marvel at the complexity and efficiency of our feet and take extra care of them. The feet are the body's shock absorbers. They each withstand the force of one and a half times our body weight when we walk. The average person takes enough steps to log 1,000 miles a year. And that's just the average. Think of people whose jobs require them to stand or walk all day.

Each foot has approximately 100 working parts—26 bones, 33 joints, 17 ligaments, and 19 muscles. A fourth of all the bones in your skeleton lie in your feet.

Each toe has three bones, called phalanges (except the big toe which has only two) for a total of 14. The toes are connected to five longer bones called the metatarsals. Then come five bones in the midfoot called the tarsals, which form the arch. The hindfoot consists of the bone in the heel, called the calcaneus, and the ankle bone, called the talus. These are covered by a complex web of muscles and ligaments that allow the foot to move in a variety of ways.

Some foot problems are hereditary. Some are due to a structural defect. But a surprisingly large percentage are due to poorly fitting shoes. The right athletic shoe is especially important for avoiding overuse injuries.

ANKLE FRACTURE

What It Is

The good news is that baby boomers are more physically active than people of their age in previous generations. The bad news is that this active, older population is contributing to a rise in the number and severity of broken ankles. This isn't to suggest that anyone should turn away from lifelong exercise because of the minor risk of injury. But if you've broken your ankle, you have plenty of company.

Breaks can happen in several places. The ankle is the joint that lets the foot bend up and down. The ankle is where the leg bone, called the fibula, joins the shinbone (tibia). The knobby bumps you feel on either side of your ankle are the ends of these leg bones. Either of these bones can break, from a fall, an auto accident, or some other trauma.

Signs and Symptoms

If you break your ankle, you'll have immediate and severe pain, swelling, and bruising. You'll be unable bear weight on your foot. You will be most tender directly over the fractured bone. If the bones have not only broken but have shifted, you may notice that the ankle is deformed.

When to Call the Doctor

The symptoms of a fracture are similar to that of a severe sprain, so every ankle injury with the symptoms described above should be checked by a doctor. Failure to treat a fracture promptly can lead to post-traumatic arthritis.

How to Treat It

The doctor will X-ray your ankle to identify the location and severity of the break. You'll need to wear a leg brace or cast to immobilize the bones while they heal. You may have a cast that goes above the

When a Child Breaks an Ankle

If your child breaks an ankle, he or she should be checked regularly for up to 2 years. That's because while bones are still growing, a fracture, if not monitored after it heals, can lead to problems such as uneven leg length or a leg that has an abnormal bend.

knee at first, which can be replaced later by a below-the-knee walking cast. If ligaments are torn or if the bones are dislocated, surgery is necessary to repair the ankle. (See p 31 for information on cast care.)

It will take at least 6 weeks for the break to heal and possibly several months before you can resume playing sports. It may be necessary to keep your weight off your ankle initially, so you may have to use crutches for several weeks until you can shift to a walking cast.

ANKLE SPRAIN

What It Is

A sprain is one of the most common injuries in both children and adults. Stepping onto an uneven surface, tripping, or otherwise twisting your ankle can stretch or tear one or more of the three ligaments in the ankle (see figure on p 210). You may suffer a minor stretch with momentary pain, or you can have a more serious injury that affects multiple ligaments and will need a doctor's care.

Signs and Symptoms

You'll feel a sudden pain, and, if it's a severe strain, may even hear a pop when the injury occurs. Depending on how severe the injury, you'll have trouble moving your ankle or bearing weight. There likely will be swelling, and the ankle may bruise due to the bleeding of the torn ligaments.

How to Treat It

If the sprain is minor, take an anti-inflammatory medication such as ibuprofen for the pain and try the RICE method:

1. Avoid bearing weight on your ankle.
2. Apply ice for 20 minutes every 2 hours.
3. Wrap the ankle in an elastic compression bandage or an ankle brace.
4. Elevate your ankle above your heart for 48 to 72 hours.

With this treatment, the swelling should go down within several days. Wear a commercially available ankle brace when you start walking again to protect the ankle while it's still healing.

Acupuncture can accelerate reductions in swelling and pain.

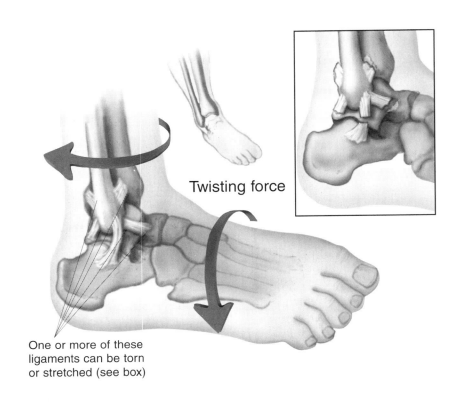

Twisting force

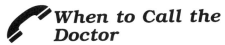

One or more of these
ligaments can be torn
or stretched (see box)

When to Call the Doctor

If the pain is severe or if the symptoms fail to improve after a few days with home treatment, call your doctor. You may need to have your ankle immobilized with a brace or a removable cast boot for 2 weeks. You'll be encouraged to put some weight on your ankle while it's protected, as this can help the healing. After the period of immobilization, you doctor will prescribe exercises to strengthen the muscles and ligaments and increase your flexibility. These may include ankle curls or standing on your toes, then your heels (see figures pp 211-212).

Eventually, you can resume normal walking or even jogging with your ankle in a brace or taped. A severe strain can take up to 3 months to heal.

Rehabilitation is important because if you don't strengthen the ankle with exercise, it's vulnerable to being injured again or sustaining permanent damage. Your ankle could develop arthritis or become unstable, putting you at risk for fractures.

Surgery is rarely needed for an acute ankle sprain. Repeated sprains may mean the ligaments are stretched out and need to be tightened surgically.

Prevention

✔ If you've had one sprain, you're at risk for another. Slow down if you feel pain or fatigue in your ankle, and exercise to keep your muscles strong and flexible. Be sure to wear sturdy shoes.

Ankle Strengthening Exercises

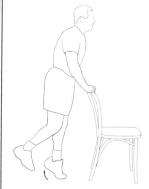

Calf Raises

Stand on a flat surface, with your weight evenly distributed. Hold the back of a chair or onto a wall for balance. Raise the heel of your uninjured leg off of the floor as high as you can, using your body weight as resistance. Work up to 3 sets of 10.

Ankle Curls

Sit on a chair or on the edge of a bed so your feet don't touch the floor. You can also lie flat on the floor. Pull your toes toward you and then push them away from your body. Repeat for 2 to 3 minutes at a time, two to three times a day.

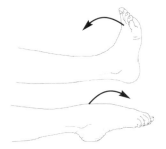

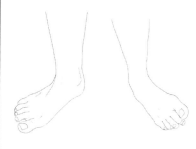

Eversion/Inversion

Sit on a chair or on the edge of a bed so your feet don't touch the floor. You can also lie flat on the floor. Slowly move your foot from side to side. Repeat for 2 to 3 minutes at a time, two to three times a day.

ACHILLES TENDON INJURIES

What It Is

? The strongest and largest tendon in the human body takes its name from Greek mythology. Achilles was a mighty warrior with only one weak spot—his heel. During a Trojan War battle, he was killed when an arrow pierced it. The Achilles tendon connects the heel bone (calcaneus) with the calf muscles in the lower leg.

Being the body's strongest tendon, able to withstand forces of 1,000 pounds or more, doesn't prevent it from being injured. In fact, it is the body's most frequently ruptured tendon because it takes a pounding during sports or running. It's especially common among weekend exercisers who try to do too much too fast. Failing to stretch and warm up before exercising, running more

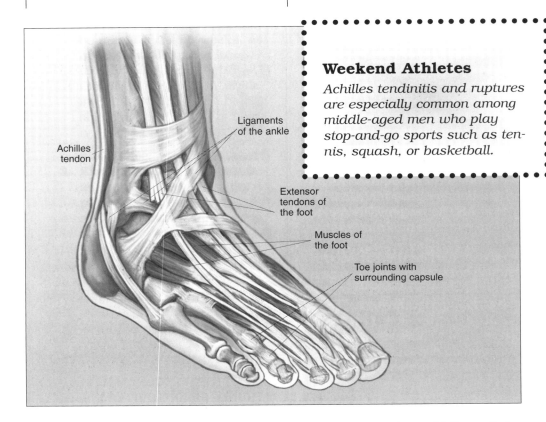

Achilles tendon

Ligaments of the ankle

Extensor tendons of the foot

Muscles of the foot

Toe joints with surrounding capsule

Weekend Athletes

Achilles tendinitis and ruptures are especially common among middle-aged men who play stop-and-go sports such as tennis, squash, or basketball.

miles than usual, or playing extra sets of tennis is a prescription for injury. Even well-conditioned athletes can suffer tendinitis or a tendon tear (rupture) if they modify their routines too much. Changing playing surfaces, such as switching from running on an indoor to an outdoor track, or wearing new running shoes can cause problems, too.

Signs and Symptoms

If you've merely strained the tendon, causing the irritation known as Achilles tendinitis, you'll notice mild pain after exercising. When you get up in the morning, you may have tenderness about an inch and a half above the spot where the tendon attaches to the calcaneus. If you fail to treat the injury, the pain will gradually worsen and may be noticeable during exercise or a few hours later. There may also be stiffness in the leg and swelling around the tendon. If it is very inflamed, the back of the leg over the tendon will feel warm to the touch.

If the tendon ruptures, you'll experience sharp, sudden pain and swelling from the calf muscles to the heel. Without treatment, your leg may become weak and you may have trouble walking. Oftentimes, people mistakenly believe that they've simply sprained their ankle, which is why these symptoms need to be checked out by your doctor.

How to Treat It

If you start to experience mild pain, rest your foot for a week. Skip your normal exercise routine, or switch to something else, such as swimming, that won't aggravate the sore tendon. Apply ice for 20 minutes several times a day for the first 3 days to relieve pain and reduce swelling. Take anti-inflammatory pain medication such as ibuprofen. Wearing a well-cushioned athletic shoe will help decrease stress on the tendon. Once the symptoms go away, don't repeat your exercise mistakes or you could face long-term consequences.

Shoe inserts such as heel pads also can help reduce stress on the tendon. Other treatments include deep-heat ultrasound, massage, and stretching exercises to strengthen the leg muscles.

Sometimes surgery is necessary to repair a torn Achilles tendon. You may have to wear a cast afterward, and you may need physical therapy to prevent muscle weakness.

When to Call the Doctor

If the symptoms don't go away after you've rested your foot for a few days, or if the pain is severe, call your doctor. Other conditions such as heel bursitis have similar symptoms, so it's important to see a doctor for a proper diagnosis.

Prevention

✔ Choose running shoes with adequate cushioning in the heel. (See p 234 for tips on buying athletic shoes.) If your heel bone is poorly aligned, a prescribed orthotic (insert) for your shoe can help position it properly.

When you exercise, be sure to warm up first and cool down afterward. Give special attention to stretching and strengthening your calf muscles. If you want to increase your running or your distance, do it gradually, in increments of 10% a week. Avoid strenuous sprinting or hill running if you haven't worked up to it.

ATHLETE'S FOOT

What It Is

❓ You don't have to be an athlete to get this itchy skin condition, but it's especially common in people who play sports. Athlete's foot is caused by a fungus that thrives in warm, damp places, such as the floors of locker rooms, and feels right at home in sweaty shoes and socks. It's most common in teenagers and men.

Signs and Symptoms

You'll notice persistent itching and a rash, usually between the toes and on the sole of the foot. If left untreated, the infection may progress, turning into blisters and watery discharge

or peeling and cracking skin. It can also spread to other parts of the body such as the groin area (jock itch) through contact with your towels, bedding, or hands that have touched the feet.

How to Treat It

Athlete's foot is a stubborn skin condition that can be hard to get rid of. Early detection and treatment helps. Try applying over-the-counter antifungal medications, all of which come in lotions, ointments, powders, and sprays. Keep your feet as dry as possible, both to inhibit the growth of the fungus and to prevent future outbreaks.

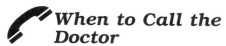

When to Call the Doctor

Call if home treatment doesn't work in 3 to 4 weeks. Your doctor can prescribe stronger medications, both topical and oral, to clear up the infection.

Prevention

Keep your feet dry by changing your socks regularly and wearing shoes that breathe.

BUNIONS AND BUNIONETTES

What It Is

A bunion is a bony knob that protrudes from the base of the big toe (see figure, left, below). If you have it on one foot, you'll likely have one on the other. It's mainly a problem for women—only one in 10 suffer-

ers is a man. Adolescents, especially girls ages 10 to 15, may develop bunions, too. The tendency to develop bunions runs in families, but the main culprit is a shoe that is too tight. High heels are a contributor, too, because they force the toes deeper into the toe box of the shoe.

Bunionettes, sometimes called tailor's bunion, are similar to bunions except that they appear

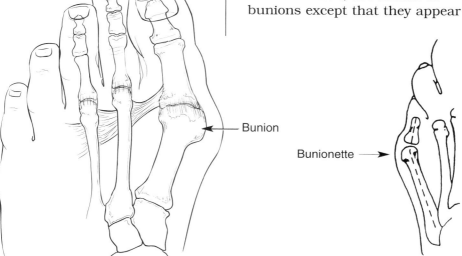

Bunion

Bunionette →

on the opposite side of the foot near the base of the little toe. Here, too, tight shoes are the main cause (see figure, right, p 215).

Signs and Symptoms

At first, the bunion looks like a small bump, and it may not hurt. But the bigger your bunion gets, the more painful it is for you to wear shoes, especially tight ones. The friction from the bulge rubbing the inside of the shoe can cause bursitis, a painful inflammation in the fluid-filled sac that develops over the bump. If you have bursitis, the area will be red and swollen and may even feel hot to the touch.

The big toe may start to angle toward your second toe or even move all the way under it, forcing the second toe out of alignment and giving the foot a distorted appearance (see figure below). You may even develop arthritis in the toe if the condition is allowed to progress.

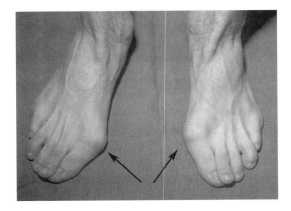

Another sign of a bunion is the distortion of your shoes. As the knob grows, it forces the shoe leather out. As the bunion gets worse, finding shoes you can wear comfortably becomes increasingly difficult.

How to Treat It

The simplest solution to easing the pain of an early-stage bunion is buying wider shoes that don't put pressure on it. Avoid high heels. Shoes with soft uppers and no thick stitching over the bunion are best. You may also need to have a shoe repair shop stretch the spot that will cover the bunion.

When to Call the Doctor

Call if changing to more comfortable shoes doesn't relieve the pain. The doctor may recommend other steps, including arch supports to decrease pressure on the bunion if the shape of your foot is contributing to the problem.

If nonsurgical treatment fails to relieve the pain when you walk, there are several surgical procedures to correct bunions that can usually be done on an outpatient basis. The doctor shaves down the bunion and realigns the bone to prevent recurrence. You can usually bear weight on the foot within a few weeks of surgery.

Dressings are changed at the doctor's office weekly for 4 to 8 weeks, depending on the severity of the bunion. Athletic or walking shoes can be worn 4 to 8 weeks after surgery, and you can resume wearing regular shoes by about 3 months.

Surgery is not recommended for adolescents, except in extreme cases. Since the bones haven't fully formed, there is a strong probability that the problem could recur.

Prevention

 Wear shoes that are slightly wider than your foot. (See p 234 for buying advice.)

CLAW TOE

What It Is

A claw toe looks exactly like it sounds. The toes curl up and then under, much like an animal claw (see figure). If you have one or two claw toes, the cause can be poor fitting shoes, but if all toes are affected, especially if both feet are involved, the condition is more likely the result of some neurologic disorder that weakens the foot muscles and creates imbalances, causing the toes to bend. Diabetes and alcoholism are two diseases that can lead to claw toe. Injury to the foot can also cause the problem.

Signs and Symptoms

 Usually all the toes are involved. They bend upward from the joints at the ball of

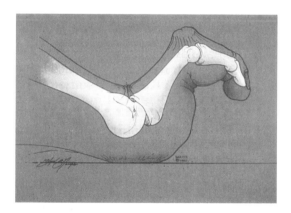

the foot and downward at the middle joint. Sometimes the end joints bend down so that the toes dig into the soles of the shoe and form painful corns on the tips. Wearing shoes becomes painful. Corns may form over the top of the toe or under the ball of the foot.

How to Treat It

Usually, this condition doesn't respond to home treatment. However, if only one or two toes are involved, you can try metatarsal pads to relieve pain in the ball of the foot. If you have corns, you can try a corn pad. Often, though, home treatment doesn't help.

When to Call the Doctor

Call if all your toes are involved or if you have pain that isn't corrected with home treatment. If you catch the problem in the early stages, your doctor may be able to correct it with splints or tape that hold the toes in the correct position. After treatment, you can help prevent the toes from curling again by using your hands to stretch the toes into their normal position and holding them for 5 seconds. Repeat two or three times each day. You can also perform foot exercises with your toes such as picking up marbles or crumpling a towel laid flat on the floor. These exercises strengthen the toes and keep the joints from becoming stiff.

Cushioning pads can help relieve the pain of corns and take the pressure off so they shrink.

If the condition has already progressed to the point where your toes won't bend out of the claw position any more, you may be able to get pain relief by buying shoes with a roomy enough toe box or have your shoes stretched to accommodate the deformity. Buy shoes made of soft material so they stretch easily. You can also wear a metatarsal pad that redistributes your weight, thus relieving pressure on the ball of your foot. If the pad helps but you want a more permanent solution, an alternative is a custom-made orthotic. (See p 238 for more information on orthotics.)

Surgery can correct the problem if these other measures fail to provide relief from discomfort.

Prevention

Wearing properly fitting shoes can prevent a claw toe from developing in some cases, but not when the claw toes are the result of a medical condition such as a neurologic disorder.

CORNS AND CALLUSES

What It Is

? Calluses aren't necessarily a bad thing. If you've noticed a callus on your finger where your pen rests, for example, that build-up of skin helps pad the bone at a spot where you apply pressure when you write. Calluses on the feet build up for the same reason. They look a bit like yellow candle wax and usually don't hurt. Calluses tend to form on the bottoms of the feet as a result of friction caused by the foot sliding back and forth inside a shoe that is too loose.

Corns develop as the result of shoes that are too tight, putting pressure on the toes. Sometimes the cause is a seam or stitching inside the shoe that rubs the toe. Even poorly fitting socks can cause corns. Certain toe deformities such as claw toe and hammer toe can also be responsible for the formation of corns. (See pp 217 and 229 for detailed information on these conditions.)

Signs and Symptoms

Hard corns are usually located on the top of a toe or on the side of the little toe. As the surface layer of the corn gets hard, it pushes on the softer tissue underneath and can become quite painful. It will look

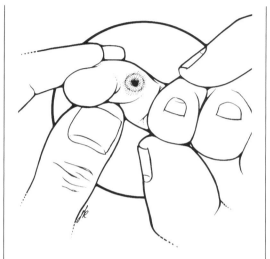

like a bump and have a tender spot in the middle surrounded by yellowish dead skin.

Soft corns look more like open sores, and they are found between toes where the toes rub together (see figure). Usually corns only hurt when you apply pressure to them.

How to Treat It

Soak your feet regularly to soften the corns and calluses and then use a pumice stone or callus file to remove the dead skin. To ease the pain of a hard corn while you have your shoes on, try wearing a nonmedicated, donut-shaped foam pad over the corn to cushion it from pressure.

If you have a soft corn, use a bit of lamb's wool or a foam spacer between the toes to cushion them. Don't use cotton because it mats down too quickly and loses its cushioning effect.

You can also try an over-the-counter corn remover, but follow the directions carefully and don't use it longer than recommended because it can harm your skin.

. . . .

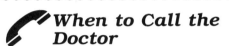

When to Call the Doctor

If home treatment doesn't relieve your pain and you can't wear your shoes, see your doctor. He

can treat the problem and also determine if you have an underlying problem such as a toe deformity that requires correction.

The doctor can reduce the corn by shaving off the dead layers of skin with a scalpel, something you should not try at home. If the problem is a toe deformity, outpatient surgery can correct it.

Prevention

Wear shoes and socks that fit and give your toes plenty of room.

Diabetic Foot Care

Foot problems that are minor for most people can become major emergencies if you have diabetes. Because one of the complications of the disease is nervous system impairment, you can lose feeling in your feet. Therefore, you won't necessarily feel an injury such as a cut, corn, or blister. Additionally, you may have poor circulation so injuries take longer to heal, making you more vulnerable to infection. Compounding the problem, infections spread more rapidly in people with diabetes.

Check Your Feet Daily

Diabetic foot problems are a common cause of hospitalization and amputation. The best way to avoid problems is to take good care of your feet and to examine them every day so you can catch problems early.

Diabetic Foot Care (continued)

Inspect your feet for swelling, bruises, pressure areas, redness, warmth, blisters, scratches, cuts, puncture wounds, corns, athlete's foot, and nail problems. A mirror can help you see the bottom of the foot. Don't forget to check between your toes.

If you find anything wrong with your feet, no matter how slight, don't try treating it yourself. See your doctor.

Never use drugstore medications such as corn removers or antiseptic solutions on your feet nor any sharp instruments or heating pads. Don't put your feet in front of a fireplace or on radiators because you may not detect when they are too hot. Wear loose socks to bed and don't get your feet wet and cold in snow or rain. In winter, wear warm socks. Avoid smoking as it decreases the blood supply to your feet.

Advice on Shoes and Socks

Don't walk barefoot or wear sandals or thongs because of the risk of injury. Buy shoes that are comfortable and don't need breaking in. Opt for shoes that breathe, such as those with leather in the upper part. Don't wear the same pair of shoes every day. Give them 24 hours to dry out after wearing. Check inside each shoe before putting it on and don't lace them too tightly or too loosely.

Put on clean, dry socks each day. Don't wear them if they have holes or wrinkles. Avoid socks with elastic tops as they can inhibit circulation.

Foot Care Do's and Don'ts

1. *Wash your feet daily with mild soap and water but don't soak them because that can dry them out.*

2. *Test the water temperature first so it's not too hot.*

3. *Pat each foot dry, don't rub it.*

4. *Apply lotion to keep your feet soft and moist, but don't put any between your toes.*

5. *Trim your nails straight across, not curved, and not too short. This prevents ingrown toenails. If you have trouble seeing or reaching your toenails, see your doctor for trimming.*

Flatfeet and High Arches

What It Is

? Babies and toddlers appear to have flat feet when they are standing because their feet have fat pads. A slight arch may appear when the child sits or stands on tiptoes. Children are born this way; doctors refer to it as flexible flatfoot. Usually it's painless and doesn't interfere with a child's ability to walk or play sports. Most children outgrow it eventually as their feet get larger, their baby fat disappears and their foot muscles strengthen with weight-bearing activity such as walking.

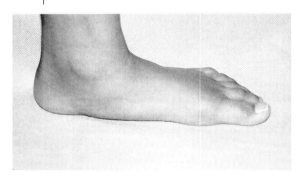

Signs and Symptoms

Although painless in young children, flatfeet in older children and adolescents can cause an aching pain. Sometimes the pain only occurs during or after sports or other physical activity. Sometimes the child complains that his foot, ankle, or leg is "tired" and that he has aching pain at night. If the Achilles tendon (at the back of the ankle) is involved, it may become red and painful. Sometimes there are calluses under the sagging arches.

When to Call the Doctor

Call if your child complains of foot pain, if the ankle is red, the feet or ankles feel tired, or calluses are forming under the arches. Be sure to take your child's shoes along to your appointment so the doctor can examine the pattern of wear. Adolescents who still have flatfeet and complain of pain should also be evaluated by a doctor.

How to Treat It

Treatment may include stretching exercises to lengthen the heel cord (see figure). Your doctor may also recommend shoe inserts called orthotics. These custom-molded arches made of composite materials provide support and relieve pain. Shoe inserts not only help people with flatfoot to walk comfortably, they also extend the life of their shoes, which otherwise would wear unevenly.

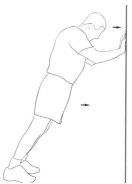

Heel Cord Stretch

Stand 3 feet from the wall with your feet pointed straight ahead. Lower your hips to the wall without raising your heels off the floor. Hold for 5 seconds. Repeat 3 to 6 times.

In certain cases, physical therapy is recommended, and sometimes children are put in casts if the heel cords are too tight. In a few cases where other treatments don't relieve pain, surgery is recommended.

Prevention

The tendency to have flatfeet runs in families, although there can be other causes as well. It can't be prevented.

High Arches

Just as feet with low arches can cause problems, so can feet with high arches, sometimes called cavus foot. A high arch is sometimes seen in children but may not be noticed until adulthood. As with flatfeet, high arches sometimes are hereditary.

People with high arches are vulnerable to overuse injuries during sports and exercise because their feet aren't good shock absorbers. Not as much of the foot touches the ground to provide support for walking.

Custom-molded shoe inserts are prescribed for this condition. The inserts position the foot properly and provide shock absorption.

FOOT AND ANKLE ARTHRITIS

What It Is

? If your foot or ankle starts to hurt for no apparent reason, the last thing you might think of as the cause is arthritis. But it's actually a common problem as people age. Wear and tear causes the cushion of cartilage between the bones to degenerate, allowing the bones to rub together. This is called

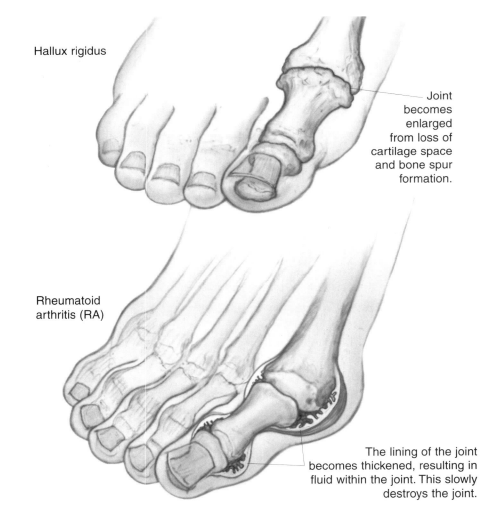

Hallux rigidus

Joint becomes enlarged from loss of cartilage space and bone spur formation.

Rheumatoid arthritis (RA)

The lining of the joint becomes thickened, resulting in fluid within the joint. This slowly destroys the joint.

osteoarthritis (OA) or degenerative arthritis, and it most commonly affects the weight-bearing joints.

Does the pain seem to be in the joint of your big toe where it attaches to your foot? That's called hallux rigidus, a type of OA that is the second most common problem of the big toe, sometimes called the great toe. (The number one problem is bunions.)

Middle Age Problem

Hallux rigidus affects approximately 2% of the population between the ages of 30 and 60 years.

Another type that can affect the foot and ankle is rheumatoid arthritis (RA). This is a disease of the joint linings that causes the lining to swell and become inflamed, and the joint space to narrow. Gradually the disease destroys bone and soft tissue. With this type of arthritis, other joints will likely be affected too, but you may notice it at first in the small joints of the feet. Women are three times more likely to have it than men, and RA can start at any age.

A third type is post-traumatic arthritis, which develops after a foot or ankle injury that doesn't heal perfectly. Most ankle arthritis is the result of trauma.

Signs and Symptoms

Arthritis pain typically develops gradually and progresses over time as the joints deteriorate. It may be worse when you get up in the morning or after you've been resting during the day. With ankle arthritis, you may notice swelling. RA usually affects more than one joint and usually affects both feet. It sometimes causes nodules (bumps) to form under the skin near the joints and also can lead to foot deformities (see figure below).

If you have hallux rigidus, you'll notice pain in the toe and stiffness that make it difficult to bend the toe upward. It can hurt more as you push off with your toes when you walk. You may also develop a bump on the top of your toe above the joint, which could become red and irritated if it rubs against the top of your shoe.

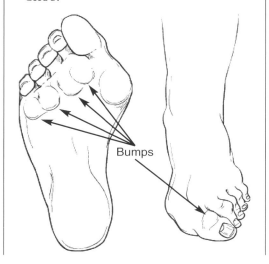

Bumps

When to Call the Doctor

Any of the symptoms above should prompt a call to the doctor since even home treatment will be more effective under a physician's guidance. Also, the doctor needs to rule out other possible causes of your symptoms.

Contrast Baths

One recommended treatment for foot and ankle inflammation (that also works for hands) is called a contrast bath.

You'll need two buckets, one filled with cool water containing a few ice cubes. Fill the second bucket with warm water (around 104°F {40°C}).

Soak the painful area for 30 seconds in the cold bucket first and then immediately in the warm bucket for another 30 seconds. Then go back to the cold bucket and alternate for a total of 3 to 5 minutes.

One easy way to do this is to take the cool bucket into the shower and alternate the cool water and the warm shower water.

Always start and end in the cold bucket. It's best if you can do this routine three times a day, but if not, soak once in the morning and once in the evening.

How to Treat It

OA can be effectively treated with various measures, including anti-inflammatory medications, ice or contrast baths to reduce swelling, shoe modifications, shoe inserts (See p 238 on orthotics.) to provide extra cushioning or support, and injections of corticosteroids.

Various surgical techniques can relieve arthritis symptoms that don't respond to other treatments, particularly RA, which can cause deformities.

If you have hallux rigidus, wear a shoe with a big toe box that won't press on the joint. Your doctor might also recommend a custom orthotic or a stiff-soled shoe with a rocker attachment. Give up your high heels, at least for a while. Anti-inflammatory pain medications and ice can reduce the symptoms as can contrast baths. Surgical treatment can help by removing the arthritic portion of the joint, or in severe cases, by fusing the painful joint so that it no longer bends. Eliminating the joint's movement removes the cause of the friction and pain.

Ankle arthritis may require the use of an off-the-shelf or custom-molded brace. Multiple surgical options are available if the symptoms persist, including removal of the debris and arthritic portions of the joint, fusion of the joint, or a total ankle replacement.

Prevention

Post-traumatic arthritis can be prevented if you seek prompt treatment of foot and ankle injuries and avoid repeated ankle sprains. Doctors don't yet know how to prevent other types of arthritis.

FOOT FRACTURES

What It Is

With 26 bones in the foot, there are a lot of places where a fracture can occur, some more troublesome than others. A heel fracture, for example, needs immediate treatment, often with surgery. A broken little toe, on the other hand, can heal with little or no treatment. Here's a brief description of what can break and what to do about it.

Heel Fracture

A fracture in the either of the two bones of the hindfoot (calcaneus in the heel and talus that sits atop it) usually occurs only with a severe trauma such as an automobile accident or a fall from a height. The symptoms are acute pain, swelling, tenderness, and an inability to bear weight. Heel fractures are serious injuries and need immediate attention. Surgery often is needed to reposition the bones.

Fractures of the Metatarsals

The metatarsals are the long bones that connect with the toes. Metatarsal fractures will usually heal without surgery. The fracture results from a direct blow—something heavy dropping on your foot or getting hit during a contact sport, for example. You'll notice pain when you bear weight on the foot and also some swelling.

Your doctor will immobilize the bone to allow it to heal. The type and degree of injury will determine the type of device you'll have to wear. They range from short leg casts or braces to shoes with wooden soles. Healing typically takes 6 weeks.

Broken Toe

If you stub your toe while walking in bare feet and it swells and turns a vivid shade of black and blue or purple, chances are you've fractured your toe bone (phalange). The most common victim is the little toe. Fortunately, this type of fracture is usually simple to treat. The broken toe can be taped to the toe next to it to keep it immobilized while it heals. A piece of gauze placed between the two toes will help absorb sweat and keep the skin from becoming irritated. The gauze should be changed daily. Only in rare cases is a broken toe injured severely enough to require surgery to reset it.

FOOT ODOR

What It Is

Some euphemisms for this problem are sweaty feet syndrome and malodorous feet. But no matter what you call it, having smelly feet can be downright embarrassing. The main cause is excessive sweat, which can be caused by emotional stress. The skin of the soles of the feet contains as many as 3,000 small sweat glands, so it's no surprise that your feet get damp!

What happens is that the climate in your shoes can become very hot and moist, causing normally occurring bacteria to grow rapidly. The growth produces a substance called isovaleric acid that gives off an odor.

It's Hot in There

Although normal body temperature is 98.6° F, the temperature inside your shoes can reach 102°F.

How to Treat It

Good hygiene is the key. Change your socks at least once a day. Also, wash your feet frequently and dust them with absorbent powder. Don't wear the same pair of shoes 2 days in a row. This allows the shoes time to dry out thoroughly between wearings.

Odor neutralizing shoe inserts may help temporarily, but ultimately, they just mask the problem.

Some people find soaking their feet weekly for 30 minutes in strong black tea is helpful. The tannic acid in the tea kills bacteria and closes pores so they don't sweat as much. Boil two tea bags in a pint of water for 15 minutes, add 2 quarts of cool water, and then soak the feet in the cool solution. Alternatively, you may use a soak made from one part vinegar to two parts water.

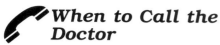

When to Call the Doctor

If your foot odor persists for longer than 4 weeks, despite home treatment, you may have a mild bacterial or fungal infection. An infection is best treated by a doctor who can prescribe oral and topical medications.

Prevention

Along with good hygiene, footwear is a consideration. Buy extra pairs of shoes so that you can let one pair dry for 24 hours after you've worn them. Make sure you buy shoes made of materials that "breathe." Leather does, for example, but synthetic materials don't.

HAMMER TOE

What It Is

If you notice that when you stand barefoot, your second, third or fourth toe stays bent at the middle joint instead of lying flat, that's called a hammer toe. Most often it's the second toe that's affected, especially if it's longer than the big toe. A bunion that pushes the big toe sideways into the second toe can contribute

to a hammer toe deformity. Rarely, a traumatic injury to the foot is the cause.

Mallet toe is similar except that the bend is in the joint nearest the nail.

As with so many other foot problems, poorly fitting shoes are often a contributing factor. If the front of the shoe is too short or

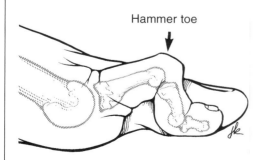
Hammer toe

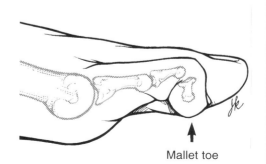
Mallet toe

narrow, or if you wear high heels that increase the stress on the toes, the toe muscles can't stretch out and eventually, you can't straighten your toe even when you are barefoot. Bottom line: The goal is for the shoe to approximate the shape of the foot, rather than for your foot to take on the shape of the shoe.

Signs and Symptoms

Besides the bent joint, a toe with either of these deformities usually has a corn on top of the bend, adding to your discomfort.

How to Treat It

Initially, the toe will still be flexible and can be easily treated. But if you ignore it, the toe can become fixed in that position and can be corrected only with surgery.

Buy shoes that are at least a half inch longer than your longest toe and are soft enough to accommodate any misshapen toes. It's also possible that a shoe repair shop can stretch your shoe to accommodate the deformed toe. Sandals may be an option, too.

Toe exercises can help stretch and strengthen the muscles. Try picking up marbles with your toes. Or crumple up a towel under your feet while you read or watch television.

When to Call the Doctor

Call if your toe doesn't improve after treating it yourself with shoe changes and exercises. Also, talk to your doctor right away if you think you have a hammer toe and you have poor circulation or numbness in your feet or if you have diabetes.

Your doctor may recommend you try commercially available straps, cushions, and nonmedicated corn pads. If all these methods fail to correct the deformity, outpatient surgery can.

Prevention

The more you wear poorly fitting shoes, the more potential there is for poor foot health. (See p 234 for tips on proper fit.) You can wear high heels provided you save them for special occasions and don't wear them to work.

HEEL PAIN

What It Is

? If you have heel pain, technically called plantar fasciitis, you are in good company. It is the most common cause of foot pain, affecting millions of people each year. Standing or walking is difficult because your heel hurts. You'll notice it especially when you get out of bed in the morning and when you stand after sitting for long periods. What's happened is that the fascia, a tough band of tissue that connects your heel bone to the base of your toe, has become inflamed.

Joggers or exercise walkers are at risk, particularly those with tight calf muscles that limit how far they can flex their ankles. Being overweight is another risk factor. Women are more likely to have plantar fasciitis than men.

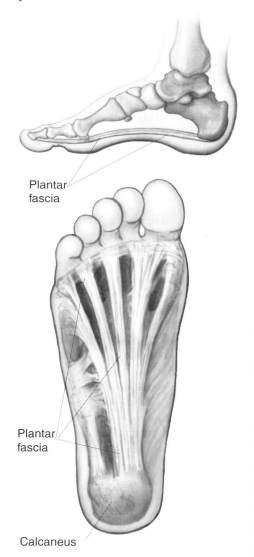

Plantar fascia

Plantar fascia

Calcaneus

What if I Stepped on a Rock?

If the pain began after you stepped on a hard object such as a rock, you may have what's called a stone bruise. You may be able to see the discoloration of the bruise, but it's not always visible. If you rest the heel, the pain will gradually go away in several days.

The good news is that in 95% of people with this condition, the pain goes away without surgery, although it may take 6 months or more for the symptoms to completely disappear.

Signs and Symptoms

It begins with mild pain under the heel bone. Typically you'll feel the pain after you exercise, not during it, which is why some people are tempted to keep jogging or walking, even though they should be giving the foot a rest.

A long-standing case of plantar fasciitis can also result in a heel spur or calcium deposit forming on the underside of the foot. It looks like a bony protrusion. The heel spur, however, is not the source of the pain. Approximately 20% of the people who have never had heel pain have heel spurs.

How to Treat It

The key to treatment is performing exercises that stretch the Achilles tendon and the plantar fascia. To help relieve the pain, apply ice for 20 minutes three or four times a day

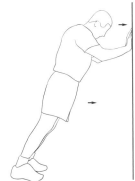

Heel Cord Stretch

Stand 3 feet from the wall with your feet pointed straight ahead. Lower your hips to the wall without raising your heels off the floor. Hold for 5 seconds. Repeat 3 to 6 times.

and take ibuprofen or another anti-inflammatory pain medication. Also, wear shoes with shock-absorbing soles, and try over-the-counter heel pads that fit in your shoes.

When to Call the Doctor

If your pain is severe or doesn't respond to home treatment in 6 to 8 weeks, call your doctor, who can recommend additional measures. Without treatment, your gait may change and cause problems with your knee, hip, or back.

The doctor may inject the heel with a corticosteroid. You might need to wear a splint when you sleep to keep the plantar fascia and Achilles tendon stretched out.

But I Still Want to Exercise

You don't have to give up exercise while recovering from plantar fasciitis. Just pick a routine that doesn't put pressure on the heel, such as swimming or riding a stationary bike.

Prevention

There is no evidence that a program of stretching exercises will prevent the condition, but stretching is good for your foot and ankle in general so it's worth the effort.

If the Shoe Fits—A Buying Guide

Bet you never thought of shoes as a public health problem! Ill-fitting shoes are a key reason one in six people have foot or ankle problems. Americans incur billions of dollars a year in treatment costs and lost work time because they don't buy shoes that fit properly.

When you forgo comfort for style, you may be contributing to a range of problems such as bunions, corns, calluses, and hammer toes. Women with a preference for high heels are especially vulnerable. It's not just the height of the heel that's the problem. High-heeled shoes frequently have pointed toe boxes that force the toes to be pushed into a triangular shape. Buying shoes that are too narrow to comfortably accommodate the width of the foot is a common mistake women make in the name of fashion.

The higher the heel, the more pressure there is on the ball of the foot as it is forced into the pointed toe box. There's also the risk of twisting an ankle while teetering on high heels.

Buying Comfortable Shoes

Okay, so style is important to you. But that doesn't mean you can't combine fashion with foot health. Consider, too, that shoes that fit well aren't causing unsightly bunions, corns, and calluses that can make your feet unattractive when you are barefoot.

If you are a woman who loves high heels, you don't have to give them up altogether. Just save them for special occasions such as an evening on the town when you are only going to be wearing them for a few hours.

Here are some tips for safe shoe shopping:

1. Go shopping at the end of the day. Your feet swell after a day of sitting and standing, so you should have shoes fitted when your feet are at their largest.

2. Ask the clerk to measure both feet every time you buy shoes. Your foot size gets larger as you get older.

3. Try on both shoes to make sure they are comfortable since most people have feet that vary slightly in size. Then buy shoes that fit your larger foot. The shoe should be a half inch longer than your longest toe.

Buying Comfortable Shoes (continued)

4. Walk around in the shoes to get a better idea of how comfortable they are.

5. Don't buy shoes that are marked in your size without trying them on. Sizes can vary among brands or even styles within a brand.

6. Stick with heels no higher than 2¼", whether they are ladies' pumps or men's cowboy boots.

7. Check to see that the shoe fits your heel as well as your toes. Your foot shouldn't be sliding in and out of the heel, and you should be able to freely wiggle all your toes.

8. Backless shoes and sandals, which are so popular today, are not good for extended walking because you have to strain your toe muscles to keep them on your feet. It's better to buy sandals with a strap behind the ankle to hold them in place.

9. Shoes with softer soles that provide more cushioning tend to be more comfortable, especially if your job requires you to stand for long periods. Shoes with softer uppers can stretch to fit the foot rather than force the foot to conform to the shape of the shoe.

10. Forget about "breaking-in" periods. The shoes should fit as soon as you put them on. If they are tight, don't buy them. Too much space isn't good either, because your foot could slide around inside the shoe and develop blisters.

Remember that the goal is to buy a shoe that conforms to the shape of your foot, not make your foot conform to the shape of the shoe!

Buying Athletic Shoes

Shoes are the most important part of an athlete's equipment. Whether you are running, hiking, playing soccer, or taking an aerobics class, the correct shoe can make the difference between comfortable exercise and painful injuries. The correct shoe will even enhance performance. Socks are important too, because they absorb shocks and prevent blisters caused by skin rubbing against the shoe.

The kind of shoe you need depends on the exercise or sport you participate in. Shoes designed for exercise walking, for example, have a smooth tread that encourages the natural roll of the foot during the walking motion. Shoes for runners have soles with deeper treads for traction but

Buying Athletic Shoes (continued)

which can impede walkers. Shoes for court sports such as tennis or vol-leyball are made to support quick movement of the body forward, backward, and side to side. Some manufacturers offer a variety of cross-trainers that work in more than one activity. With all the types to choose from, it's a good idea to consult a knowledgeable salesperson in a sporting goods store for the type that best serves your needs.

Field sports such as soccer, baseball, and football require cleated shoes. Your coach can advise you on what type to buy.

But I Love My Old Tennis Shoes

One of the biggest mistakes people make with athletic shoes is continuing to use them when they are wearing out and offer less protection. If you walk or run regularly, buy a new pair at least every year and more often if you run more than 10 miles a week.

How to Find the Right Athletic Shoe

1. *Try on athletic shoes after a workout and at the end of the day when your feet are largest.*

2. *Wear the same kind of socks you exercise in when you try on the shoes.*

3. *Note especially if the shoe has wiggle room for the toes and that it grips the heel rather than allowing it to slip.*

4. *Check that it has good shock absorption.*

5. *Walk or run a few steps to further check for comfort. Remember: don't plan to break them in.*

6. *Remember: Shoes should fit immediately.*

7. *When your child's new sports season starts, remember to check that the shoes he or she wore last season still fit.*

Buying Athletic Shoes (continued)

Surprisingly, how you lace your athletic shoes can help a lot to improve fit. Shoes with a larger number of eyelets will make it easier for you to get a custom fit. In general, you should loosen the laces before you slip your foot into the shoe, then, starting with the eyelets closest to your toes, tighten one set at a time.

Here are some specific foot problems and lacing techniques to accommodate them.

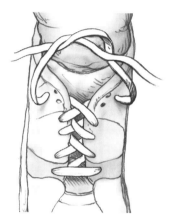

Narrow Feet

Use the eyelets farthest from the tongue in order to bring up the sides of the shoe.

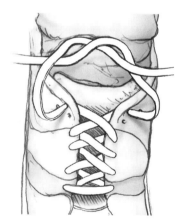

Wide Feet

Use the eyelets closest to the tongue to give the foot more space.

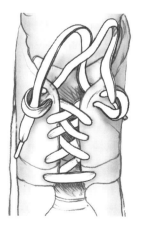

Heel Problems

Use every eyelet, making sure that the area closest to the heel is tied tightly. Put less tension on the lacing near the toes. When you reach the next to the last eyelet on each side, thread the lace through the top eyelet making a small loop, then thread the opposite lace through each loop before tying it.

Buying Athletic Shoes (continued)

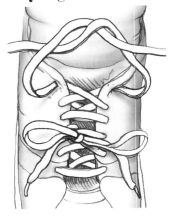

Narrow Heel and Wide Forefoot

Use two laces. Thread one through the top half of the eyelets and the other lace through the bottom half. Tie the laces in the top half—closest to the heel—more tightly than the bottom one.

Buying Orthotics

If you have particular foot problems such as high arches or heel pain, special inserts, called orthotics can help. You may be able to benefit from inserts sold over-the-counter. But for more difficult problems, your doctor may suggest you have inserts custom-made to fit the shape of your foot and provide the extra support you need.

Buying Children's Shoes

When your baby starts to walk—usually around the first birthday—that's the time to buy shoes. Until then, booties or socks to keep her feet warm are all you need. Once she's walking, she'll need shoes for outside, but it's fine for her to walk barefoot inside.

Kids' Feet Sure Do Grow

Children's feet grow fast so check their shoes regularly to see if they are getting snug. The younger the child, the faster his feet will grow. Early on, expect to buy a new pair at least every 2 to 3 months. By the time the child is 3 years old, the intervals may stretch to 6 months. One sign that a toddler's shoes may be getting too tight is if he frequently takes them off or if they cause him to trip.

Buying Children's Shoes (continued)

When you buy your baby's first pair of shoes, it's best to go to a children's shoe store, if possible, because it will have a wide selection of sizes and styles, and the clerks should be more knowledgeable about fitting toddlers. Most pediatricians recommend comfortable shoes with nonskid soles such as sneakers. High-topped shoes with ankle support are not necessary.

The sales clerk will check to make sure there's enough room in the shoe for the toes to wiggle. There should also be about a finger's breadth of space at the end of the shoe toe for the foot to grow. Don't be tempted to buy a larger size that your child will be able to wear longer because a shoe that is too large can contribute to falls or may cause sore spots on the foot where it slides around.

Avoid Using Baby Walkers

Baby walkers, those devices on wheels in which babies can stand or sit and propel themselves around, actually hinder children learning to walk rather than help them. The leg muscles don't develop as quickly because the walker allows the baby to get around so easily. What's worse, walkers have caused thousands of broken bones and other serious injuries because babies fell down stairs in them. Bottom line: don't use a walker.

INGROWN TOENAIL

What It Is

An ingrown toenail can develop if you cut your nails too short, causing the corners of the nail, most often on the big toe, to dig into your skin. It also can be the result of wearing shoes that are too tight.

It's not only painful, but you risk developing an infection.

Signs and Symptoms

At first your toe feels very sore and may be swollen. If the pressure continues or if you pick at it, the toe can become infected and turn red. You might even see pus drain from around the nail.

How to Treat It

Soak your foot in warm, soapy water two or three times a day. Apply an over-the-counter antibiotic cream to help prevent infection. And if you can't wiggle your toes in your shoes easily, stop wearing them.

When to Call the Doctor

Call your doctor if the pain and redness persist after a few days. You probably have an infection. Your doctor can prescribe an oral antibiotic and instruct you on home care. In addition to soaking the toe, the doctor may suggest you insert some waxed dental floss or cotton between the nail and the skin, using a cotton

swab. Replace the packing each day. This keeps the sharp nail edge from cutting into or irritating the inflamed skin.

If you are in a lot of pain, or the infection recurs, your doctor may numb the toe and remove the affected part of the nail.

Consider wearing clean socks and open-toed shoes or sandals while the toe heals.

Prevention

Don't make the mistake of trimming your nails following the curve of your toes. Toenails should be trimmed straight across with no rounded corners. Don't trim too short, either. The nail should extend out past your skin, and not end right against the nail bed. This is especially important in people with diabetes who may have less feeling in their toes.

INTOEING

What It Is

Many parents of infants panic when they notice that their baby's toes turn inward—sometimes called pigeon toes—when walking. Usually it's

nothing to worry about, and most children will outgrow it before their second birthday. It's sometimes due to the way the infant was lying in the uterus. Some children inherit the tendency from their parents.

240

Signs and Symptoms

Usually these conditions aren't painful and don't interfere with a child's ability to walk. If the intoeing is severe, it could cause the child to trip, but that's normal for toddler even without the condition.

How to Treat It

In most cases, there is no need for treatment. In the past, doctors sometimes recommended special exercises or used braces, shoe inserts, or casts to force the feet to point straight ahead. Today we know those measures are not necessary and may even hinder the child's ability to walk.

If the child's intoeing is due to a slight turning of the lower leg bone (tibia), he or she will probably outgrow it by age 3. If it's caused by an inward turning of the thighbone (femur), it becomes most apparent when the child is around age 5 or 6. In either case, the child will likely outgrow it by around age 8 to 11.

Surgery is rarely considered even if the child still has a problem after age 9 or 10 and it's severe enough that it significantly interferes with walking. Surgery usually is recommended only when the child has intoeing associated with motor problems such as cerebral palsy.

Outtoeing and Other Abnormalities

Outtoeing

By age 2, most kids walk with their toes pointed slightly outward. If the feet angle out excessively this is called outtoeing. It isn't as common as intoeing, but in most cases, it is also just part of normal development. If you want reassurance that your child is walking normally, ask your doctor during a routine well-child visit.

Metatarsus Adductus

Some infants are born with feet that bend inward from the middle of the feet to the toes. This is called metatarsus adductus. It can resemble a clubfoot, which is a different and more serious deformity. Metatarsus adductus is a common condition that usually improves on its own. If the child reaches the age of 6 to 9 months and the condition isn't better, your doctor may recommend special corrective shoes or casts. In most cases, this treatment corrects the deformity.

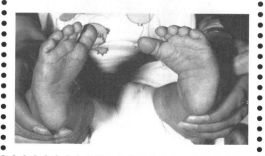

Some parents worry that letting their toddler with intoeing walk barefoot will hurt his feet. Not true. It's perfectly okay for him to walk barefoot, except when he needs shoes to keep warm or to protect his feet when he's outside.

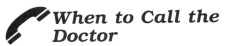

When to Call the Doctor

If you are concerned, ask your doctor about it during your child's routine well-child visit.

Prevention

✔ As kindergarten teachers have advocated for years, when kids sit on the floor, they should sit cross-legged rather than with their legs at their sides forming the shape of a W, which stretches the legs and feet into an abnormal angle.

MORTON'S NEUROMA

What It Is

? With Morton's neuroma, it feels as if you are walking around with a marble under the ball of your foot. Or maybe it feels more like there is a wrinkle in your sock.

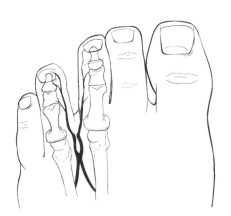

It's not really a neuroma, which is a benign tumor of a nerve. Instead, it's a thickening of the nerve between two toes caused by repeated irritation (see figure). It usually occurs between the third and fourth toes, but it can also occur between the second and third toes. Usually, only one foot is affected.

The fact that women have Morton's neuroma much more often than men suggests that narrow, high-heeled shoes contribute to the problem by pushing the toes together and irritating the nerve.

Signs and Symptoms

The key symptom is pain in the ball of the foot that may radiate into the toes. The pain worsens when you put on shoes and when you engage in physical activity. It gets better when you take off your shoes and massage the ball of your foot. The two affected toes may feel numb or otherwise uncomfortable. Since it's not really a tumor, normally you won't see a lump under your foot.

How to Treat It

Try wearing comfortable cushioned, low-heeled shoes for 4 to 6 weeks. That way, the bones can spread out and take pressure off the nerve until it heals.

When to Call the Doctor

If you still have pain after trying the cushioned shoes, call the doctor to rule out other possible causes such as a stress fracture or arthritis.

Sometimes doctors recommend pads or customized shoe inserts to lift and separate the bones. You may also need an injection of a corticosteroid medication to reduce the swelling and inflammation. Only a small number of patients need surgery.

Prevention

Wear comfortable shoes. You may also need to change your exercise program if it puts a lot of stress on your feet.

NAIL FUNGUS INFECTION

What It Is

Fungal organisms thrive in warm, moist places such as health club locker rooms and school gym showers. Nail salons that don't maintain sanitary conditions during manicures and pedicures can spread them, too. Once the organism gets under your toenails, it has found a warm, moist home in which to thrive. The stubborn infection that results can be difficult to get rid of.

Nail fungus infection is one of the few foot problems that affect more men than women, perhaps because more men walk barefoot

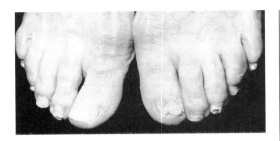

in locker rooms. Age is a factor, too. Half the sufferers are people older than 70.

Some people view it simply as a cosmetic problem and ignore it. If one person in the family has it, however, it can spread to other members who may not be as accepting of the idea of having ugly toenails.

Nail Salon Safety

Professional pedicures can transmit infections if not performed properly. Make sure the salon you go to meets the following standards.

1. *Maintains clean, sanitary conditions*

2. *Is licensed and displays the licenses—with photo ID–of each operator*

3. *Uses cleaned or single-use implements for each customer*

4. *Uses small brushes to prevent nail polish and other products from coming in contact with skin*

Signs and Symptoms

The nails will become thicker and appear to be chalky yellow or white (see figure). Sometimes the area around the nail itches. Trimming your thickening nails can become difficult. If the nails get too thick, wearing shoes can become uncomfortable.

When to Call the Doctor

This is not an easy condition to cure so rather than trying home treatment with over-the-counter medications, it's best to see your doctor. As with many conditions, nail fungus infections are easier to treat if you catch them early.

How to Treat It

The doctor will trim your nails and scale away the dead layers and may prescribe a topical medication. If the fungal infection is very far advanced, the topical medication can't penetrate the thickened nail. In that case, you can take prescription oral medications. These are very effective but must be taken for several months.

Prevention

Don't go barefoot in locker rooms and pools. If you have a pedicure, make sure the nail salon uses sterilized instruments or take your own.

PLANTAR WARTS

What It Is

Does it feel as if there's a stone in your shoe but there's nothing there? You may have a plantar wart, which appears on the plantar or sole of the foot and is caused, as are all warts, by a virus that enters the body through a break in the skin. The virus grows in warm, moist environments, so you're more vulnerable if you walk around a locker room in your bare feet or your feet sweat and the moisture is trapped in your shoes. It's particularly common in children and teenagers.

Signs and Symptoms

Unlike the kind of wart you get on your finger or elsewhere, plantar warts grow into the skin rather than protrude out. That's because of the weight you put on your feet when you stand or walk, which pushes the wart inward.

Appearance-wise, you might confuse this wart with a callus which looks a bit like yellow candle wax and is found over weight-bearing areas of the foot (figure, left). A plantar wart tends to be in a non-weight-bearing area and typically has some tiny black dots on the surface (figure, right). These dots are the ends of small blood vessels, not found in calluses. Also, you won't see normal lines or "fingerprint pattern" of the skin on the area where the wart is.

The wart can be very tender if you squeeze it from side to side, and that's another way to distinguish it from a callus, which won't hurt if squeezed sideways. Sometimes plantar warts multiply into clusters called "mosaic warts." Or, one wart will spawn a few surrounding "babies." Plantar warts can also spread to other parts of the foot and grow larger.

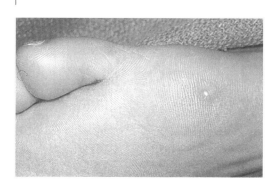
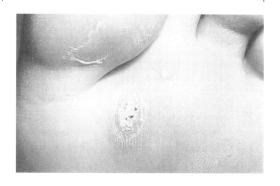

How to Treat It

Most warts go away by themselves in 5 or 6 months. But many are tricky to get rid of. If yours does not appear to be disappearing on its own, nonprescription salicylic acid patches or "wart sticks" available in drug stores can help dissolve warts. Multiple applications are needed, and it may take weeks for the wart to completely disappear. In between applications, you can rub the wart with a pumice stone to remove the outer layers of dead tissue. Just be careful that you confine the treatments to the wart itself and not the surrounding tissue, as it can be damaged by the acid and the pumice stone. Be sure to wash your hands thoroughly after treating a wart to avoid spreading it to other areas!

Caution: Don't use home wart removers if you have diabetes. (See p 220 for information on care of the diabetic foot.)

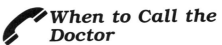

When to Call the Doctor

Call if the wart is painful, especially large, or otherwise bothersome. Under a doctor's supervision, you can try stronger topical medications.

If that doesn't work, your doctor may recommend removing it by freezing the tissue with liquid nitrogen. Freezing can only be done to the top layer of the wart so this procedure typically takes several sessions until the wart is dissolved. Some warts respond to an injection of medications. Your doctor may try a laser treatment. In rare cases, doctors recommend surgery to cut out the wart.

Prevention

To avoid picking up the virus, wear shower shoes or sandals when you use a public locker room or shower. Keep your feet dry by changing your socks frequently and using foot powders.

STRESS FRACTURES

What It Is

? A stress fracture is a tiny crack in the bone caused by repetitive overload. Ankles and feet are prime locations for such overuse injuries because they take the biggest hit when you walk or run. People who suddenly begin a serious walking or running program without gradually building up to it are prime candidates for stress fractures. So are people who quickly increase the intensity or distance of their exercise or who switch from running on soft surfaces to hard surfaces. Even your athletic shoes can cause the problem if they are too worn out to give you proper support or if they don't fit right.

The most common spot for a stress fracture is the metatarsal bones, which are the long bones connected to the toe bones.

Signs and Symptoms

As with other types of fractures, pain and swelling are common, but the symptoms develop more gradually and are less severe than with a fracture due to a direct blow. The pain gets worse as you bear weight on your feet, and it is relieved by rest.

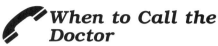

When to Call the Doctor

If you have these symptoms, call the doctor so the severity of the fracture can be assessed. An examination will show tenderness and swelling directly over the site of the fracture. The doctor may not order X-rays because if they are taken within 2 weeks of the beginning of symptoms, the stress fracture usually doesn't show up. Later, X-rays may show it when the bone is healing.

How to Treat It

In most cases, stress fractures will heal if you reduce your activity level. If the break is in a metatarsal bone, you may be advised to wear a stiff-soled shoe, wooden-soled sandal, or removable short leg walking cast. Certain types of breaks may require you to wear a cast and use crutches.

Prevention

Build up gradually when you exercise, and make sure your athletic shoes provide adequate support. Replace them regularly and buy new ones that fit from the start with no "breaking in" period. (See p 234 for buying advice.)

TOE WALKING

What It Is

You may think you've got a budding ballet dancer in the house. Lots of children walk on their tiptoes when they first begin to walk. They usually stop doing it, however, in a few months. But toe walking in children past 18 months of age is called habitual toe walking, and treatment may be needed.

Signs and Symptoms

Toe walking can vary in severity. The child usually can stand with feet flat on the floor and can walk using the full foot if reminded. Some may not be able to move their ankles up and down fully.

When to Call the Doctor

If your child is still walking on her toes 6 months after she first learns to walk and doing it more than 90% of the time, let your doctor know. Also, call if the child walks on only one toe as this could indicate a neuromuscular problem and should be checked out.

How to Treat It

Older toddlers who only walk on their toes occasionally just need observation. Sometimes stretching exercises are prescribed. Children who are older than 3 years and still persist in toe walking may need to wear a series of casts or day and night braces that reposition the ankle muscles. The child may also need a physical therapy evaluation to assess whether she has any sensory or motor problems. Physical therapists can also perform exercises to stretch the heel cord and instruct parents on doing these exercises at home. A shoe that positions the ankle and foot, particularly for a toddler, may be recommended, too. In a few cases, with older children, surgery is needed to relax the heel cord.

Prevention

Early diagnosis and treatment can help prevent toe walking from becoming a more serious condition.

TURF TOE

What It Is

As artificial turf increasingly covers athletic fields, there's been a rise in sprains of the toe joint nearest the ball of the foot, commonly dubbed turf toe. But it can happen on a hard court, too. If you are crouched down and roll with force onto your toes so they bend more than normal, the ligaments stretch and may tear. In nearly all cases, it's the big toe that is affected. It's a common injury for soccer or football players and others involved in high-speed sports.

Signs and Symptoms

Swelling, tenderness, or severe pain and limited motion in the first joint of your toe (where the toe meets the ball of the foot) are common. Depending on the severity of the sprain, there may be bruising, and you won't be able to walk normally.

How to Treat It

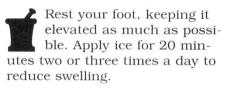

Rest your foot, keeping it elevated as much as possible. Apply ice for 20 minutes two or three times a day to reduce swelling.

When to Call the Doctor

Call if there is little or no improvement after about 48 hours of home treatment or if the pain is severe. The doctor will immobilize the foot in a walking cast or a postoperative type shoe for 1 or 2 weeks, and you'll have to stop playing sports for 4 to 6 weeks while it heals.

Prevention

Other than giving up your sport, there's nothing you can do to prevent turf toe.

NECK AND SPINE

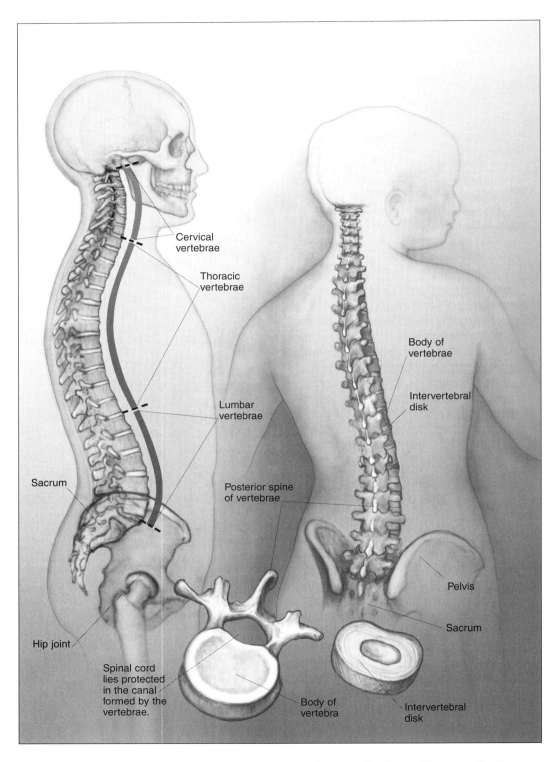

Cervical
vertebrae

Thoracic
vertebrae

Lumbar
vertebrae

Sacrum

Posterior spine
of vertebrae

Hip joint

Spinal cord
lies protected
in the canal
formed by the
vertebrae.

Body of
vertebra

Body of
vertebrae

Intervertebral
disk

Pelvis

Sacrum

Intervertebral
disk

NECK AND SPINE

THE SPINE IS A COMPLEX structure of bones and soft tissue with several important jobs. It supports the upper body, protects the spinal cord, absorbs shocks, and allows us to bend.

In this chapter we'll explain what can cause neck and back problems, how they are treated, and how to prevent them. First, it's helpful to understand the spine's structure and how it works.

Your spine is actually a line of bones called vertebrae that stretch from the base of your skull to your buttocks. The vertebrae are connected by tough bands of tissue called ligaments. In between the vertebrae are disks, cylindrical pads that cushion the bones and act as shock absorbers when you move. A disk has a hard outer layer and is gel-like inside.

No two vertebrae are shaped exactly alike, but doctors group them according to location. The top seven are the cervical, or neck, vertebrae that hold up your head. Next are the 12 thoracic, or chest, vertebrae that are shaped so they'll join with the ribs. The five bones in the lower back are the lumbar vertebrae. At the bottom are the five vertebrae that make up the sacrum, which joins the pelvis or hip bones, and the coccyx, also called the tailbone.

The vertebrae form a protective, vertical tunnel that houses your spinal cord, which, along with the brain, makes up the central nervous system. The spinal cord carries messages from the brain to other parts of the body. The vertebrae also have holes along their sides to accommodate bundles of nerves about the diameter of your little finger, which run from the spinal cord to other parts of the body and provide a path for signals from the brain. Near the tip of the spine, several nerves combine to form two sciatic nerves, which branch apart and run down either side of the body into the hips and legs. They are the largest nerves in the body and are sometimes the source of a common type of back pain called sciatica.

Various groups of muscles are also attached to the spine. They provide support and flexibility to the spine and make movement possible. If you keep your back muscles strong and flexible through exercise, you'll be a lot less likely to suffer from back pain.

"BURNERS AND STINGERS"

What It Is

? A common neck injury in athletes is called a "burner" or "stinger." It's a weird sensation, sort of like the feeling when you hit your funny bone. An athlete—youth or adult—takes a hit that affects the neck and causes a tingling pain or numbness down the arm, sometimes all the way to the hand. The injury usually occurs when an athlete's head is forcefully pushed sideways and down, bending the neck and causing the nerves to be pinched or compressed. Stingers and burners are most likely to happen in contact sports such as football and wrestling.

Signs and Symptoms

You are likely to feel a shock-like or tingling pain or numbness that starts at one shoulder and proceeds down the arm. The reason the sensation feels as though it can "travel" all the way from the neck to the fingertips is because the roots of the nerves that control the arms and legs are in the neck. In some cases, partial paralysis, weakness, or loss of sensation can occur.

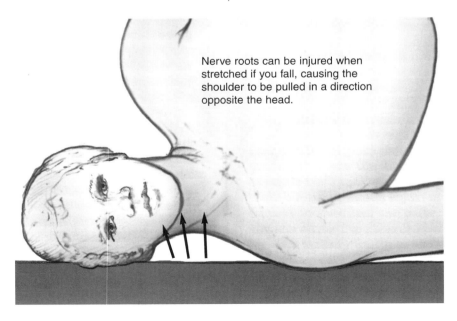

Nerve roots can be injured when stretched if you fall, causing the shoulder to be pulled in a direction opposite the head.

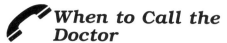

When to Call the Doctor

In most cases, the pain or sensation in the arm and hand will go away in a few minutes. If strength in the arm and hand don't return after that time, call your doctor. Also call if this is a recurring problem.

How to Treat It

First, stay out of the game until the symptoms have gone away. If the symptoms don't subside quickly, the doctor will recommend rest to reduce the pressure on the nerves. Also, take an anti-inflammatory medication such as ibuprofen to reduce swelling and relieve pain. As the pain or numbness subsides, you can gradually start some simple neck strengthening exercises.

Along with rest and medication, the doctor also may recommend other treatments. You may be told to wear a soft cervical collar, for example, to keep your neck from bending during the healing process.

Prevention

In a contact sport, getting hit goes with the territory. You may not be able to do much to prevent burners and stingers except to keep up with neck strengthening exercises. There's a lot you can do to prevent sports injuries in general, however. (See p 22 for information.)

CHRONIC NECK PAIN

What It Is

If you injure your neck, in a fall for example, you'll likely have an acute (sudden) pain. But if you have wear-and-tear (arthritic) changes in your neck that develop gradually, there may be pressure on a nerve root that leads to chronic neck pain, also known as cervical radiculopathy. No matter what it's called, it can really hurt!

The most common causes of this condition are the following.

1. **Herniated cervical disk.** Disks are pads that act as cushions between vertebrae. If the firm outer layer of a disk cracks or wears out and the gel-like center breaks through, the disk can protrude and put pressure on the nearby nerve where it exits the spinal column.

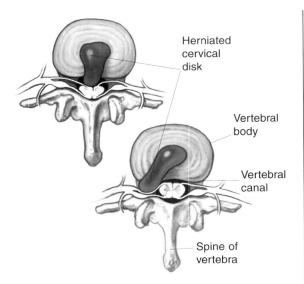

Herniated cervical disk

Vertebral body

Vertebral canal

Spine of vertebra

2. **Spinal stenosis.** This condition occurs when the space in the center of a vertebra narrows and squeezes the spinal column and nerve roots.

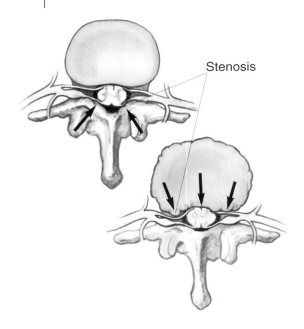

Stenosis

3. **Degenerative disk disease.** The aging process takes its toll on the body. The water content in our cells diminishes and other changes occur that can make the disk and cartilage shrink. That leaves the vertebrae without enough padding, causing them to press against each other and pinch or press on a nerve. Bony spurs may form, too. Typically, this occurs in people older than age 40.

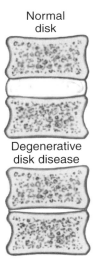

Normal disk

Degenerative disk disease

4. **Inflammatory diseases.** Osteoarthritis, which usually affects older people, and rheumatoid arthritis, which can affect people of any age, may damage the joints in the neck, causing pain and stiffness.

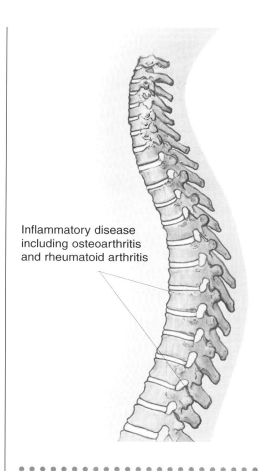

Inflammatory disease including osteoarthritis and rheumatoid arthritis

When to Call the Doctor

Call the doctor if your neck pain is severe or if it is continuous for more than 48 hours. Also, seek medical attention if your pain radiates down the arms or legs or is accompanied by headaches, numbness, tingling, or weakness lasting more than 48 hours.

How to Treat It

Initially, your doctor may advise rest and anti-inflammatory medication such as ibuprofen to relieve inflammation and swelling. You may also be advised to wear a cervical collar to limit motion and relieve irritation on the nerves. Some physical therapy may also be needed such as heat or cold therapies, electrical stimulation, or use of a cervical traction device, which looks like a stiff collar and is available in retail stores.

If these treatments don't relieve your pain in about 6 to 12 weeks, surgery may be needed. In most cases, it not only stops the pain but also improves your ability to move your neck.

Prevention

Keeping fit through regular exercise may prevent some neck problems. Also, make sure your body is positioned properly when you perform work that requires you to hold your head in one place for long periods, such as working at the computer.

KYPHOSIS

What It Is

? When you were young, did your parents nag you to "Stand up straight"? If you have children, you've probably echoed this plea. All this nagging and pleading stems from worries parents have that their children will develop a rounded or hunched back from constantly slouching. Some curve in the spine is normal as viewed from the side (figure, left). Kyphosis is the term used when the curve is exaggerated (figure, right). It is typically seen in adolescents.

Signs and Symptoms

Postural kyphosis, or a rounded back, usually develops during adolescence and is more common among girls than boys. It seldom causes any pain, and most teens grow out of it as they age and their posture improves.

A less common condition but one that also occurs during the teen years—and more often in boys than in girls—is Scheuermann's kyphosis. It affects the child's appearance but is seldom painful. When it is, physical activity or long periods of standing or sitting

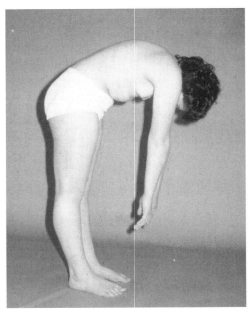

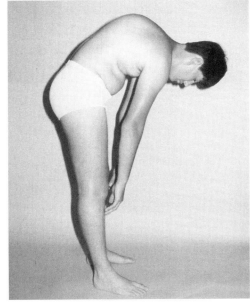

can aggravate pain. With this condition, the upper (thoracic) spine is usually affected.

In both conditions, the child's back has a rounded appearance. The way the two are distinguished is through X-rays. Scheuermann's kyphosis is identified by distinctive appearance of the vertebrae.

When to Call the Doctor

If your child complains of back pain, you should call the doctor. But it's also reasonable to call if you, or your child, is worried about the appearance of a rounded back. The doctor may order an X-ray to measure the degree of the curve. A curvature, as viewed from the side, greater than 50° is considered abnormal. An X-ray can also identify if there are any bone abnormalities such as with Scheuermann's kyphosis, where the vertebrae are irregular and wedge-shaped.

How to Treat It

Treatment depends on the reason for the abnormal curvature. With postural kyphosis, your doctor may suggest an exercise program at home to help improve your child's posture by strengthening the abdomen and stretching the hamstring muscles. Your doctor or a physical therapist will show your child how to perform the exercis-

Adult Spines Can Curve, Too

Older adults can have rounded or humped backs, too, but not for the same reasons as adolescents. It's likely due to a condition such as osteoporosis that weakens the bones, causing them to press on each other.

es. A common exercise recommended for this condition is simply lying flat on a firm floor.

For teens with Scheuermann's kyphosis, initial treatment can include an exercise program plus anti-inflammatory medications and rest if pain is a symptom. If your child is still growing, the doctor may have him wear a brace until the spine matures. A brace can stop the progression of the curve and even improve it. In the rare cases of extreme curvature, corrective surgery may be needed.

Prevention

Stay physically fit. Teens who spend long hours sitting in front of their computers should be reminded to stand up and stretch occasionally or lie down on their backs on a firm surface (such as the floor) for a few minutes.

LOW BACK PAIN

What It Is

? If your lower back hurts, you're in good company. Back pain is the second leading cause, after colds, of visits to the doctor. Four out of five adults experience a significant episode at some point in their lives. Sometimes it's caused by lifting a heavy object the wrong way. People with jobs requiring frequent bending and lifting are particularly at risk. Your back, which is designed for movement, also may stiffen if you sit for hours at a desk. Other contributors include poor posture, being overweight, smoking, stress, and pregnancy.

The wear and tear of aging can cause low back problems, too. The strength and elasticity of muscles and ligaments diminish with age, joints stiffen, and bones weaken. There may be degenerative changes in the disks or arthritic conditions in the joints. If these conditions become severe, they can cause stiffness and pain. Although you can't stop getting older, you can slow the effects of aging on your back by staying physically active and fit.

Signs and Symptoms

Pain centered in your lower back can develop slowly or may appear suddenly. It may start after you lift something

Stand Up Straight!

1. *Good posture puts less stress on the back, so don't slouch when you stand or sit.*

2. *If your job requires you to sit for long periods, get up and move around every hour or so.*

3. *If your chair doesn't support your lower back, try using a pillow made for this purpose.*

4. *Wear low-heeled shoes.*

5. *Sleep on a mattress with firm support.*

6. *Shed some pounds if you are overweight.*

7. *Don't smoke (it harms your blood vessels and seems to increase the risk of back pain).*

Backpack Safety Checklist

Does your child look like a beast of burden? It's common to see young-sters weighed down with heavy packs on their backs, toting a musical instrument case in one hand and sports equipment in the other.

It's the backpack that has parents and school administrators worried. Can a load this size cause poor posture or even back injuries?

Although there is little risk of serious damage, children can suffer muscle fatigue and back discomfort from carrying heavy backpacks. They may even develop bad posture habits such as excessive slouching.

An informal, nonscientific survey of 100 members of the American Academy of Orthopaedic Surgeons and the American Academy of Pediatrics in 1999 found that 58% had seen young patients complaining of back or shoulder pain from their backpacks. Your child can do a few simple things to prevent this problem:

1. ***Position the Load.*** Make sure the backpack is positioned properly. Your child should be using both straps, not slinging the pack over one shoulder. Adjust the straps so the backpack is held firmly in place, about 2" above the waist. Place the heaviest items closest to the back.

2. ***Pack Light.*** Some kids carry extra weight needlessly because they don't consider which books they really need to carry home from school and just bring them all. Encourage your child to visit her lock-er frequently to replace books and, at the end of the day, to pack only those that are needed for homework. Some families purchase extra books so their children can leave one set at home and one at school. Remind your child to clean out the backpack periodically to eliminate old term papers, broken pencils, dirty gym shorts, and other excess baggage. You'd be surprised how much that will lighten the load!

3. ***Buy the Right Backpack.*** Choose a smaller pack over the jumbo size. If your child has limited space, she'll be forced to consider more carefully how much she really needs to cram into it. Make sure that the backpack has padding on the back and wide, padded straps. Get one with a hip strap and encourage your child to use it for heavy loads. In some schools, backpacks with wheels are catching on.

> ## Use Your Legs, Not Your Back
>
> 1. *It's important to lift and move objects properly to avoid back pain.*
> 2. *Position the object close to your body before lifting it.*
> 3. *Plant your feet a shoulder width apart.*
> 4. *Lift with your leg muscles, not your back.*
> 5. *Lower your body by bending your knees, pick up the object, and then raise yourself up with your legs, keeping your back straight.*
> 6. *Don't twist your body; point your feet, and pivot your body in the direction you want to move.*
> 7. *Get help if an object is too heavy or is so awkwardly shaped that it can't be controlled easily.*

or after a fall. But it also can develop for no apparent reason. It may be so severe that you are unable to move.

How to Treat It

Most cases of low back pain aren't serious and respond to simple treatments. Years ago, doctors advised complete bed rest but not any more. Even though you'd probably prefer to lie still until the pain goes away, you'll recover faster if you can ease into light activity such as walking as soon as possible. You may have to modify your normal work or recreational activities for a while.

Take anti-inflammatory medication such as ibuprofen, both to ease the soreness and to reduce the inflammation. Applying ice packs for 20 minutes every hour or so can relieve the pain, too. Don't apply ice directly to the skin as this can cause frostbite.

Spinal manipulation (as done by a chiropractor) or acupuncture has been shown to ease back pain. No such evidence exists for magnets and other alternative treatments. Because some cases of back pain can be caused by our response to stress, techniques such as yoga or meditation can be helpful.

When to Call the Doctor

Call if the pain lasts for 3 or 4 days and hasn't responded to any of the recommended treatments. Call also if the pain is severe and occurred due to an injury, or if you have recurring episodes of back pain. The doctor will also want to know if the pain radiates down into your hips or legs, as this could be a sign of sciatica. (See p 161 for information on this condition.) In some cases, the doctor may order imaging tests of the bones and soft tissues to help with the diagnosis.

In rare cases, back pain can be a sign of a serious medical problem. Consult your doctor if the pain is accompanied by fever, rapid weight loss, or bladder control problems, if it interferes with sleep, or if you have a history of cancer.

Prevention

✔ Get moving! The best way to prevent back pain is to keep the muscles strong and flexible. Stay active by biking, walking or swimming, for example. Conditioning exercises are important, too, as they work specifically

---

At Risk for Back Pain?

Caregivers for ill or injured family members are at special risk for back pain. Pulling a bedridden person into a sitting position, or helping a person move from the bed to a chair puts extra stress on the back. So does carrying a toddler or lifting him into his car seat or high chair. The tips on proper lifting apply whether you are moving an object or a person. Don't be in a hurry; plan ahead; and remember to bend your knees and let your leg muscles do most of the work.

---

to strengthen and stretch the back, hip, thigh, and even the stomach muscles. A strong abdomen helps you stand straight.

NECK SPRAIN

What It Is

? A ligament sprain—or muscle strain—can be a real pain in the neck. Sprains can occur during sports, a fall, or a car collision for example. (See p 270 for information on whiplash.) The neck is especially vulnerable to injury because it is less protected than other parts of the spine. The good news is that unless the injury is severe, neck

pain is usually a temporary condition that will disappear over time with proper treatment.

Signs and Symptoms

You may feel the pain immediately after the injury, or it may develop gradually and peak a day or two after your injury. You may experience one or more of the following symptoms:

1. Muscle spasms in the upper part of your shoulders
2. An ache at the back of your head
3. Numbness, weakness, or tingling in the arms
4. Increased irritability
5. Fatigue
6. Difficulty sleeping and concentrating

You may also have stiffness, and you may not be able to move your head very far from side to side, up and down, or in a circular motion.

How to Treat It

With mild pain and no other symptoms, take an anti-inflammatory medication such as ibuprofen. You can also apply an ice pack for 15 to 30 minutes several times a day for the first 2 or 3 days after the injury. Applying heat, especially moist heat, for about 20 minutes at a time helps loosen cramped muscles, but you shouldn't do this until about 72 hours after the pain started. That's because heat generates more blood flow to the affected area and can cause swelling. Return to normal activities as soon as your comfort level improves. Mild aerobic exercise, such as walking, can speed your recovery.

Some evidence suggests that spinal manipulation (as done by a chiropractor) or acupuncture has

been shown to ease neck pain. No such evidence exists for magnets and other alternative treatments. Because some cases of neck pain can be caused by our response to stress, techniques such as yoga or meditation can be helpful.

Caution: *Athletes who suffer a cervical sprain should not return to play until the symptoms are gone and they have full range of motion again. Check with your doctor or team athletic trainer for clearance to return to play.*

When to Call the Doctor

If the pain lasts longer than 3 or 4 days or if it is severe enough that ibuprofen doesn't provide some relief, call your doctor. You should also call if you have symptoms other than neck pain such as numbness or pain that radiates down your arms or legs.

Depending on the diagnosis, the doctor may prescribe muscle relaxants to ease spasms and may also recommend that you wear a soft cervical collar for a week or two to help support your head and relieve pressure on your neck while it heals. A cervical pillow available from stores that sell medical supplies may help you sleep more comfortably during the healing process. Your doctor may also suggest isometric exercises or physical therapy as your comfort level improves during the first 2 weeks. Massage and ultrasound are sometimes prescribed if the pain is severe.

Prevention

Always wear your seatbelt in the car. To prevent sports injuries, you should exercise all your muscles, including your neck.

SCOLIOSIS

What It Is

If you stand behind your child and look at her back, her spine should be like the letter "I"—a straight line down the middle. Children with scoliosis have spines that curve from side to side. On an X-ray, the scoliosis spine looks more like a letter "S" or a "C" (see figure). We don't know what causes it, but we do know that it runs in families.

Signs and Symptoms

In children, scoliosis tends to develop before puberty, and it's rarely painful. Beginning when your child is about 8 years of age, watch for these signs:

1. Uneven shoulders
2. Prominent shoulder blade (one or both)
3. Uneven waist
4. Elevated hips
5. Leaning to one side

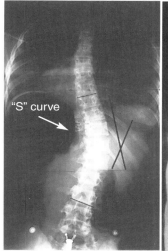
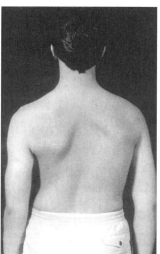

"S" curve

Many schools have scoliosis screening programs so your school nurse also may alert you to these signs.

When children are somewhere between 8 and 10 years old, most family doctors and pediatricians begin routinely checking for scoliosis during annual physical exams. The child is asked to bend

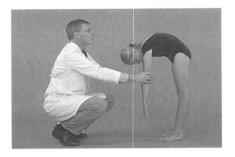

forward with arms hanging free
and feet together, making the
bones more visible (see figure).

When to Call the Doctor

If you notice any of the above
signs, call your doctor who will
order an X-ray to measure the
curve. In most cases, the curve
will remain small, and the child
simply will be checked periodically to make sure the curve isn't
getting larger.

Look at and Listen to Your Daughters

*Scoliosis is seven times more
likely to occur in adolescent
girls than in boys. The reason for this gender difference
is unknown. If your daughter
(or son) complains that her
"clothes don't hang right,"
that might be a tip off that
she needs to be checked for
scoliosis.*

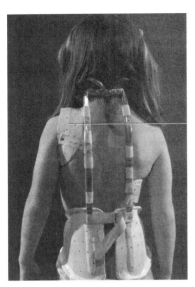

How to Treat It

If the curve gets larger or
progresses, your doctor will
prescribe a brace to prevent
further progression (see figure).
But don't worry. A child with a
brace can still play sports and be
physically active.

In a few cases—if the scoliosis is
severe when it is first diagnosed
or if the brace doesn't control the
curve—surgery may be necessary.

Prevention

Good posture makes for a
healthier back, but it won't
prevent scoliosis. There's
nothing you or your child can do
to prevent scoliosis. But you can
minimize the severity through
early detection. Keep an eye out
for the symptoms, especially if
there is a history of scoliosis in
your family.

Scoliosis in Adults

Although scoliosis is usually seen in young adolescents, infrequently it occurs in adults. The person may have had the deformity as a child, and it was not treated or it may have developed in adulthood, often as the result of degenerative disk disease.

Back pain is what usually drives an adult with scoliosis to see the doctor. Symptoms such as rounding of the back or leaning to the side may be more noticeable. Sometimes the person reports that he or she is "getting shorter." These deformities of aging are more likely to appear in people over age 60.

As with other types of back pain, treatment begins with pain management such as with anti-inflammatory medications, aerobic exercise such as walking, and specific exercises to improve muscle flexibility and strength. Braces don't help in the treatment of adult scoliosis. In cases of severe pain, progressive imbalance, and shape changes, surgery may be necessary.

STRESS FRACTURES

What It Is

A common cause of low back pain in adolescents who play sports is a stress fracture in one of the bones in the lower back. Called spondylolysis, this condition is seen especially in youths involved in sports such as gymnastics, weight lifting, and football, which put a lot of stress on the bones in the lower back (see figure).

Problems also can result from repetitive bending and overstretching (hyperextending) the spine. The lower back may not be able to maintain its proper position. If it starts to slip out of place, that condition is called spondylolisthesis.

Children may be born with conditions of the lower back that put them at greater risk. Girls with menstrual irregularities or who have eating disorders tend to experience bone weakening so they, too, have more risk.

Signs and Symptoms

Many people have these conditions without obvious symptoms. If there is pain,

What is a Stress Fracture?

A stress fracture, sometimes called a fatigue fracture, is a tiny crack or cracks in the surface of the bone caused by repetitive stress such as frequently bending forward or backward.

it typically spreads across the lower back and may feel like a muscle strain. Usually, the onset of pain is gradual, but it can occur suddenly when the child is bending backward.

If a vertebra has slipped out of place, the child may experience spasms that stiffen the back and radiate down the hamstring muscles. The child's posture or the way she walks may look different than usual. Bending forward will be difficult.

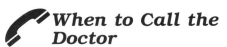

When to Call the Doctor

If your child has some of the symptoms described above, consult your doctor. Children's bones heal more quickly than an adult's, and, in most cases, the stress fracture will repair itself

with no complications or recurrence if treated promptly. Early treatment also lessens the likelihood that a slipped vertebra will progress further.

How to Treat It

The child should take a break from sports until the symptoms go away — which they often do. Anti-inflammatory medications such as ibuprofen will help ease the pain. Depending on the severity of the injury, the doctor may recommend physical therapy. A back brace might also be part of the treatment.

Prevention

To avoid recurrence of the stress fracture, the child should exercise to stretch and strengthen the back and abdominal muscles.

TORTICOLLIS

What It Is

? Torticollis is a condition, typically in infants, in which the muscle on one side of the neck is contracted, causing the head to tilt to one side and the face to rotate toward the unaffected side (see figure). The condition is also called cock-robin or wryneck. A child can be born with the condition, or it can appear in early infancy. It also can develop later as a result of a minor neck injury or a particular type of upper respiratory infection and, if it becomes severe, is called atlanto-axial rotary subluxation (AARS). AARS most commonly develops in children between the ages of 2 and 12. Very rarely, torticollis can be a sign of a tumor.

Signs and Symptoms

Along with the tilt, sometimes the face of a baby born with torticollis will appear slightly flattened on the affected side. When the baby is 4 to 6 weeks old, the parents may notice a lump or swelling in the neck muscle on the contracted side. But this mass typically disappears in a few weeks. It can be mistaken for a tumor and actually is called a "pseudo-tumor." If left untreated, the condition can cause permanent limited motion in the neck and uneven develop-

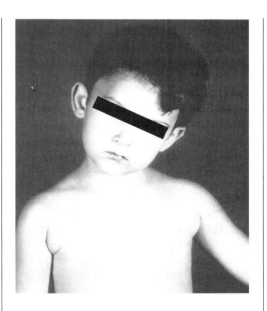

ment of the face. Sometimes children who have congenital torticollis also have hip dysplasia. (See p 144 for information about this condition.)

Children with AARS may experience neck pain, but it's usually very minor. The condition can become fixed if left untreated.

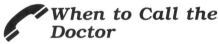

When to Call the Doctor

In most cases, your pediatrician will notice this condition during a well-child visit. If you notice your child's head persistently tilting to one side or a lump on the side of the neck, contact your doctor.

How to Treat It

For children with congenital torticollis, frequent stretching exercises that tilt and rotate the head can correct the problem. Parents may find it helpful to learn the techniques under the supervision of a physical therapist, but they'll still have to work with their baby on their own because the exercises must be performed several times a day.

Parents also can position the baby's crib and changing table so the infant is encouraged to look away from the affected side. If the condition hasn't been eliminated after 12 to 18 months of treatment, your doctor may recommend surgery.

Prevention

Babies are born with torticollis, and there is nothing you can do to prevent it. Fortunately, in nearly all cases it can be eliminated with physical therapy and exercises.

WHIPLASH

What It Is

If your car is rear-ended, the impact shoves your car forward. There's a split-second delay before your head and shoulders also move forward. Then, if you step on the brake to stop the car suddenly, your head and neck are thrown backward (see figure). All this sudden to and fro can result in a painful neck injury called whiplash. About 20% of people involved in rear-end collisions experience whiplash symptoms. While most people recover quickly, some have chronic symptoms.

Signs and Symptoms

Within 2 days of the accident, you may experience some of the following problems:

1. Neck pain and stiffness
2. Headaches
3. Pain in the shoulder or between the shoulder blades
4. Low back pain
5. Pain or numbness in the arm and/or hand
6. Dizziness
7. Ringing in the ears or blurred vision
8. Irritability, sleepless, fatigue
9. Difficulty in concentrating or remembering

How to Treat It

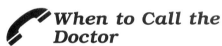 If the pain is mild and you don't have any other symptoms, take anti-inflammatory medication such as ibuprofen and apply ice to the neck area for 20 minutes, two to three times in the first 24 hours. Recovery will be quicker if you begin gentle movement, such as walking, as soon as possible. Return to your regular activities as soon as you are able, even if you have to modify your routine somewhat until the symptoms ease.

When to Call the Doctor

Call if the pain is severe or if, after home treatment, it persists while you are at rest or with each movement. Call, too, if you experience any of the other symptoms listed above such as weakness or numbness in your arms or legs, dizziness, blurred vision, difficulty concentrating, or ringing in the ears.

Doctors used to treat whiplash by immobilizing the neck with a soft cervical collar, but now the trend is to use collars intermittently and for short periods, if at all. Your doctor may also recommend isometric exercises (exercises

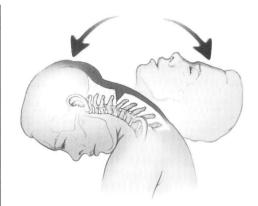

against resistance), physical therapy, massage, heat, ice, ultrasound, and medications to relieve pain. A commercially available cervical pillow may help you sleep more comfortably. Massage therapy, acupuncture, or manipulation is sometimes helpful as well.

Most symptoms resolve within 6 to 12 months. Chronic symptoms may require further evaluation and possibly surgery.

Prevention

Even if you can't avoid a rear-end collision, you may be able to escape injury if you keep your headrest adjusted to your head's height. The purpose of a headrest is to stop your head from moving very far back in the event of such a collision. And you should always wear your seat belt.

GLOSSARY OF TERMS

Acute: Sharp or severe, sudden onset, eg, pain.

Aerobic exercise: Vigorous rhythmic activity that strengthens the heart and lungs.

Arthrogram: A diagnostic technique in which dye is injected into a body structure so that the soft tissue will appear on an X-ray. The fluid either leaks into an area where it doesn't belong, indicating a tear or opening, or it is stopped from an area where it should be able to go, indicating a blockage.

Arthroplasty: Surgery in which an artificial joint is created. Also called joint replacement.

Arthroscopic surgery: Repair work done on a joint using pencil-sized instruments inserted through tiny incisions. The surgeon is guided by a fiber optic camera also inserted into the joint and connected to a monitor.

Arthroscopy: A diagnostic test in which the doctor inserts a small fiber-optic camera (arthroscope) through a tiny incision. Images from inside the body are projected onto a monitor.

Atrophy: When muscles become weakened from lack of use. For example, leg muscles enclosed in a cast to immobilize a broken ankle will be shriveled and weak when the cast comes off and will need to be exercised to restore muscle strength.

Bursae: Small, fluid-filled sacs that reduce friction between a tendon and a bone.

Bursitis: A condition in which a bursa becomes inflamed and sore from overuse.

Cartilage: The cushioning material attached to the ends of bones to cut down on friction. It can wear away with age or overuse, causing pain and inflammation.

CT scan (computed axial tomography): Used to show soft tissues more clearly than normal X-rays can, the CT scan is a noninvasive procedure that involves fraction-of-a-second X-rays that pass through a body part at different angles and then can be combined in a computer image that provides a cross-sectional view.

Cervical: Refers to the bones in the neck.

Chronic: A condition that has lasted for a long period of time, such as several weeks or months.

Compound fracture: A break in which the bone cracks and the parts move apart causing a break in the skin. Also called an open fracture.

Congenital: A condition (eg, anomaly, malformation, disease) that is present at birth.

Contrast baths: Alternately soaking the affected foot/ankle/hand in cold-water and warm-water baths.

Corticosteroids: A category of anti-inflammatory medications, including the well-known drug cortisone.

Dislocation: When a joint moves out of its proper anatomic plane.

Growing pains: A painful condition that occurs, typically in the legs, in preschool or early adolescent children. Although the cause is not known, doctors think the condition is probably related to muscle stress from overactivity such as running, jumping, and climbing.

Herniated disk: A bulge or rupture in a spinal disk.

Idiopathic pain: Pain from an unknown cause. Often used in connection with low back pain.

Joint: The place where two or more bones come together, eg, the knee or the elbow.

Laceration: A torn, ragged wound.

Ligament: Tough bands of tissue that hold bones together.

MRI (magnetic resonance imaging): A noninvasive procedure in which a machine uses a powerful magnet to produce a series of cross-sectional images of a part of the body. It is used to detect damage in soft tissues.

Muscle: A band of fibrous tissue that can contract or expand, causing the parts of the body to move.

Musculoskeletal system: The body's bones, joints, ligaments, tendons, muscles, and nerves.

Neurologist: A doctor who specializes in the diagnosis and treatment of disorders of the neuromuscular system.

NSAID (Nonsteroidal anti-inflammatory drug): Medication used to relieve inflammation and reduce pain. These include aspirin and ibuprofen.

Occult fracture: A small break in the bone that may not show up on X-rays but may be revealed on a bone scan.

Occupational therapist: A medical professional who assists people in regaining the skills of daily living (eating, bathing) and trains patients in the use of adaptive equipment.

Orthopaedist: A medical doctor with extensive training in the diagnosis and surgical and nonsurgical treatment of the musculoskeletal system.

Orthotic: A support, such as a brace, for weak or injured joints or muscles.

Osteoarthritis: Cartilage loss at the ends of bones that leads to increased friction in the joints.

Overuse injury: Repeated stress on a body part that eventually results in damage.

Physical therapist: A medical professional who helps in the rehabilitation of muscles and skeletal diseases or injuries by noninvasive means such as exercise, massage, water, heat, and electric therapies.

Prosthesis: An artificial joint.

Rheumatoid arthritis: Disease of the joint linings that causes swelling and inflammation, followed by destruction of bone and soft tissue.

RICE: Treatment method consisting of rest, ice, compression, and elevation.

Simple fracture: A break in which the bone cracks but stays aligned.

Sprain: An injury in which a ligament or a joint is weakened or torn by twisting or wrenching.

Strain: An injury in which a muscle is weakened or torn by twisting or wrenching.

Strength training: An exercise program that uses weight to keep muscles and bones strong.

Stress fracture: A tiny crack or cracks in the surface of the bone caused by repetitive pressure, such as frequently bending forward or backward. Also called fatigue fracture.

Sutures: Stitches a doctor uses to close a wound.

Synovium: Lining of the joints.

Tendinitis: Inflammation of the tendon.

Tendon: Tough bands of tissue that connect muscles to bones.

Trauma: A wound or injury.

Ultrasound treatment: Application of gentle sound waves that warm deep tissues to improve blood flow and promote healing.

INDEX

---

*Page number with *f* indicates illustration.